The Flat-Belly Kitchen:
Superfoods for a Flat Stomach

By Mike Geary, Certified Personal Trainer, Certified Nutrition Specialist
& Catherine Ebeling – RN, BSN

DISCLAIMER: *The information provided by this book, Web Site, or company is not a substitute for a face-to-face consultation with your physician, and should not be construed as individual medical advice. If a condition persists, please contact your physician. The testimonials on this Web Site are individual cases and do not guarantee that you will get the same results.*

This site is provided for personal and informational purposes only. This site is not to be construed as any attempt to either prescribe or practice medicine. Neither is the site to be understood as putting forth any cure for any type of acute or chronic health problem. You should always consult with a competent, fully licensed medical professional when making any decision regarding your health. The owners of this site will use reasonable efforts to include up-to-date and accurate information on this Internet site, but make no representations, warranties, or assurances as to the accuracy, currency, or completeness of the information provided. The owners of this site shall not be liable for any damages or injury resulting from your access to, or inability to access, this Internet site, or from your reliance upon any information provided on this site.

TABLE OF CONTENTS

PART ONE
Start the Cleanout!

PART ONE

Start the Cleanout!

By Mike Geary, Certified Personal Trainer, Certified Nutrition Specialist
& Catherine Ebeling – RN, BSN

Introduction

She's never been thin, slim, small or ever described as little. Scratch that, the ultrasound technician might've referred to her as tiny during her mother's second trimester, but that might have been the first and last time. She's always been heavy.

She's always had an inner tube around her waist. At different times in life it might be more or less inflated, but she's always had a tummy; always had a little pudge around her center. She didn't grow up lonely or depressed and always had friends. Maybe not very many, but she had them.

In middle school the only PE unit she was ever good at was the dance unit. In high school she had good, clean fun. Was voted class clown and had her first kiss sophomore year behind the bleachers. But, she was never asked to a school dance, could never share clothes with her friends, and always sat on the end of the aisles during assemblies to have enough room. She graduated high school, went to college, joined a sorority and gained the freshman fifteen. She lost the sophomore twenty and put back on the upperclassman thirty.

Through the years she indulged in all types of delicious food, going on every fad, yo-yo diet and even growing to love cottage cheese. But none of these things have made her healthier or happier with her shape for an extended period of time. The cabbage diet, cayenne pepper cleanse, and spanx might've gotten her into her prom dress for the night, but give it a few weeks and those size sixteen pants were at the front of her closet once again.

She once was worried about finding a husband, but now she has a loving husband who finds it endearing that her stomach jiggles like green Jello when she laughs. After three kids and thirteen years of marriage he's seen her at her heaviest and at her smallest. She's spent her whole life not fitting in seats as comfortably as others. Her knees always used to hit the seat in front of her, and her hips seemed to always love to flirt and cuddle with the hips of the lucky soul that was sitting next to her. It wasn't until her family went to an amusement park that she realized she needed to make a change, and fast.

Her oldest son wanted to ride one of the new roller coasters but was too afraid to ride on his own. Considering his father became light headed when he changed the batteries in the smoke detector, she knew she had to go with him. They waited in line for two and half hours to get on this ride. As they approached the front she began to feel a little nervous. Thoughts like, "*I hope I can fit in the seat. I hope I can get out on my own. I hope nobody is looking*" flew through her head. Her palms begin to sweat and she feels her face begin to flush.

They inch to the front of the line, walk around and get in their seats. Her son is seated to her right and she to his left. She pulls the harness over her shoulders and reaches between her legs to fasten herself in. She can't. The buckle is pinching her thighs, her hands begin to slip and her heart begins to sink. Her son notices she's getting a bit frustrated and tries to help. They're unsuccessful. Not wanting to ruin her son's chance at riding the ride after they'd waited so long she tries to "fake it" and simply hold the harness down in the hopes that the pimply teenager with the blonde bowl cut doesn't double check and see that she's not securely fastened. No such luck, he comes around and checks to make sure everyone was buckled and calls her bluff. Seeing how red her face had become and surely the look of desperation on her son's face he quietly tries to help them buckle her in. Failure. He discretely waves over his partner for help and the four of them, herself, her son and the two teenagers try to buckle her in. Failure again.

He leans down and whispers, "I'm really sorry ma'am. We actually can't let you ride without being buckled in and I don't think we can get it." She looks up at him, nods her head slowly, lifts the harness back over her head and gets off the ride. Her son, both scared to ride by himself and not wanting to leave his mother to walk back alone hops out of the ride too and they make their way down the exit ramp. On her walk of shame she's in shock. She's mortified, hurt, angry, embarrassed, and disappointed in herself. She spent her whole life defending her weight and trying to justify every pound that was gained and now she's come to a crossroads. Either make a change or live a life that will be forever changed and defined by the extra baggage carried around her midsection.

~~~~~~

Does this story sound like a familiar one? Can you or someone close to you relate to the feelings described in this sad and unfortunate situation? Regardless of whether this hits close to home or not, I know we all feel like we could be living and eating more healthfully.

Through recent years the rise of the so-called "healthy diet" has permeated and even bombarded our thinking. However, in one corner we hear one miracle supplement is going to change our lives, and in the other someone has found it is dangerous.

The rise of technology, and its applications in good health, medicine, and our food is actually quite frightening. The controversy surrounding the widespread availability of genetically modified foods is beginning to cause many people to question even the healthy vegetables they take home from the supermarket.

I want you to pull yourself from the confusion and the controversy, and get back to eating the simple, healthful diet of real foods our bodies were designed to consume. We are going to focus on the Nutrient Density of the food you are eating, which in turn will benefit your body and your heath in effective and potent ways.

But first let's consider one of the main methods of getting healthy and losing weight that the world has relied on for years: counting calories!

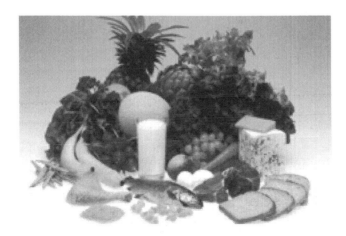

What I am about to say may surprise you, especially for a nutrition book. You can now officially STOP counting and obsessing over calories for good!

I know that sounds crazy, because it's true that calories consumed vs. calories expended over a specific time period is what ultimately controls whether you gain weight or lose weight.

However, not only is counting calories horribly inaccurate (studies show that the majority of people massively underestimate their caloric intake when asked to count calories), but also counting calories is pointless once you understand and implement one major nutrition concept. Many dieticians, nutritionists, doctors, and other health "experts" who base their recommendations on the food pyramid often overlook this principle. It's no wonder so many people are confused about nutrition!

In fact, the Nutrient Density of your food intake is the major nutrition principle and THE most important concept you'll ever need to know regarding how to eat in order to obtain great health and a lean body.

That's right... nutrient density makes calorie counting obsolete. We're talking about micronutrient density here and not macronutrient density. If virtually all the food you eat every single day is comprised of super-high micro nutrient density, then your body automatically obtains all of the nutrition it needs. Your body automatically regulates your appetite and calorie intake without you having to struggle and restrict yourself to control how many calories you eat.

Now before you think that high nutrient density only means fruits and vegetables, think again! You'll see throughout this book that high nutrient density can also include lots of high fat foods that you may have believed were "bad for you," such as whole eggs, red meat, nuts, certain oils, and butter.

Think about it for a second – If you eat foods each day that are high in calories but low in nutrients such as pasta, cakes, cookies, crackers, etc. (high caloric density, low nutrient density), then your body will be craving additional food. You may have already wasted more than your daily caloric maintenance balance for weight maintenance vs. weight gain by eating these "empty" foods.

On the other hand, if all of the foods you eat on a daily basis are super-high in nutrient density, regardless of the caloric content of those foods, your body is automatically adjusting your appetite and eliminating cravings based on it already obtaining much of the nutrition it needs for the day. This essentially forces your body to "auto-adjust" your appetite and you naturally fall within the exact caloric range that your body needs, without having to over-analyze or count calories.

In fact, eating a super-high nutrient density diet is so powerful, that extreme distance athletes who burn massive amounts of calories each day through excessive exercise may actually need to focus on consuming a portion of their diet as lower nutrient density foods, such as breads and pasta and other calorically-dense but low-nutrient foods to avoid serious weight loss.

The reason for this is that if an extreme distance athlete focuses too much of her diet on super-high nutrient density foods, her appetite may be diminished before she has eaten enough calories to sustain her massive calorie needs, and excessive weight loss may occur. Since most of us are not extreme distance athletes, this just shows you the power of eating a super-high nutrient dense diet and how you can automatically control your appetite, eliminate cravings, and get on the road to a lean healthy body for life.

In this book we're going to show you all of the low-nutrient foods that you need to avoid and get rid of, as well as some of the false "healthy" foods you've been deceived into believing were good for you. In addition, we're also going to show you all of the countless delicious options you have for healthy foods that are nutrient dense and can help to bring you closer to your goals. And I guarantee we're going to show you plenty of foods that you thought were unhealthy that can actually help you get leaner and healthier, including some tasty foods you've been lead to believe are off limits!

How to Read this Book

We're going to dig into the truth about cholesterol, saturated fats, omega 3 and omega 6 oils, fiber, protein, hormones, plant foods vs. animal foods, and tons of info that may shock you about what's actually in the food you buy at grocery stores or restaurants. You will want to begin by reading this book from front to back, so that you initially learn all the important details about what foods you should focus your diet on, and also why. It is best not to skip around this first time through, as you don't want to miss any of the important details.

Once you have read through Flat Belly Kitchen, you can keep and use this book as an everyday resource that will serve you in your daily quest to eat and live healthily. Think of this book as a companion for you and your family. The book is divided into specific sections, regarding the different food groups precisely so you can focus on the set of foods you may be working to include in your everyday diet.

Think of Flat Belly Kitchen as your new life plan for eating; your companion guide to help you navigate the crazy ideas that bombard the media each day, telling you to "eat this, not that." You now have in your hands a resource which will help you navigate into the heart of eating and preparing nutrient dense foods that come from the most natural sources possible.

Here's to your journey for true health!

CHAPTER 1
The Processing of Foods

Whether a food is processed or in its natural state has a huge impact on how your body digests and utilizes it. It also has a lot to do with whether food is stored as body fat or used for energy and rebuilding your healthy body. With all of the macronutrient debate in recent years over what type of "diet" is best for us (low-carb, low-fat, no-carb, high protein, raw, Paleo, vegetarian, vegan, etc, etc), you have to realize that they are ALL WRONG!

That's right… If you study historical dietary patterns of prehistoric humans in almost any culture around the world, the one similarity that accounted for their good health was that the foods were unprocessed and in their natural states. Whether a diet was high in protein, high in fat, high in carbs, low in carbs, etc, etc doesn't seem to matter that much, as long as the diet was made up of natural unprocessed foods, eaten as close as possible to how they are found in nature.

The general rule of thumb is that we gain weight and get fat when more calories are eaten on a regular basis than our bodies need to meet daily energy demands. When food intake is stored as fat, it is the body's natural biological response from our hunter-gatherer days.

Way back in prehistoric days, people who were able to store food in the form of fat were actually more likely to survive and reproduce during times of scarcity. Because of this advantage, we still have that built in urge to eat a lot of food when it is available, and some more than others.

The problem is that not only is there plenty of food everywhere we look, but much of it is really 'nonfood,' or just processed junk full of empty calories, fake flavorings and preservatives. Virtually NOTHING our bodies can use.

In spite of being able to store body fat efficiently, ancestral humans were rarely obese because they worked hard just to find food and shelter. In the process, they burned up whatever calories they consumed.

In the last few thousand years, we have made huge changes in agriculture and technology which has made most food easy to obtain. We no longer have to spend our days hunting and searching for food. Unfortunately most of the food that is readily available is food that our bodies do not recognize. (Until recent decades humans never ate grains to the extent that we eat them today. 70% of modern western diets are derived from grains and soy products).

One of the key reasons the food we eat gets stored as fat has a whole lot to do with the hormone insulin and our levels of blood sugar, or glucose. Insulin is responsible for keeping our blood sugar at a certain healthy level, because higher levels of glucose are extremely damaging in our bodies. When we eat foods made from processed grains, starches or sugars, including fruit juices, soda, sports drinks, breads, pasta, cookies, crackers, cake, etc., our bodies quickly turn those carbohydrates or sugar into glucose, which is used as an energy source, or stored as fat. When circulating blood sugar, or glucose goes up, insulin is secreted.

Insulin causes glucose to be transformed into fatty acids, and the body stores these fatty acids in our fat cells. So a key factor in weight gain is the presence of insulin. Insulin also causes an increase in appetite. So, that sweet or starchy snack you just ate—well, it gets stored right away as fat, AND you're hungry again in a short time. This is a vicious cycle. On the other hand, keeping your blood sugar stable, and keeping insulin levels lower, keeps your body in the fat burning zone, and that is where you want to be.

Even more importantly high blood sugar and the resulting surging levels of insulin not only make us fat, but they also make us sick. Did you realize that heart disease, strokes, cancer, diabetes, obesity, Alzheimer's, irritability, depression, ADD, arthritis, and many more diseases are often the result of high blood sugar and insulin?

So the key, then, is to purge our kitchens of those foods that cause our bodies to store fat. As we get rid of the old, unhealthy, fat-storing foods, we open the doors to transform not only our bodies but our physical, emotional and mental health as well. Revamp your kitchen and you revitalize, renew, and rejuvenate your body!

Since the days of our caveman ancestors, we were made to function best on whole, unprocessed foods, good quality proteins, healthy fats, and fruits and vegetables. If we can get back to a diet as close as possible to our ancestors, we will again have the lean, strong bodies that we strive for. Without being hungry or counting calories!

We have been duped into believing that fast, pre-made meals (diet meals) will somehow make us thin and healthy. If you check out your grocery store frozen food aisle, you will often see overweight people purchasing "diet foods." Nothing could be further from the truth!

So-called "diet foods" are chock full of fillers, extra sugar (usually in the form of high fructose corn syrup), preservatives, processed flours, soy by-products, and unhealthy fats. These "diet" or "low-fat" foods cause inflammation, stimulate the insulin response—i.e., store fat—and do nothing for you nutritionally. What's more, you GAIN weight from eating this kind of junk!

The media, the FDA, and conventional medicine have fooled us into thinking we need lots of grain-based foods to have a "balanced diet." In response America has loaded up on processed carbs and as a result, packed on the pounds and watched their health go down the drain—without ever making the connection. These "health foods" are not what our bodies recognize as good nutrition, or even as fuel for energy. And the fat-free and sugar-free options are horrible! This stuff is poison for your body, and fat storing fuel.

Forget diet foods! They take years off your life by stoking the fires of inflammation which lead to obesity and disease, not to mention screwing up your body's hormones and metabolism and making it increasingly difficult to lose fat from your frame.

If you want real "diet food" pick up a raw apple, nuts, grass-fed beef jerky, or

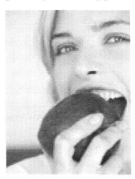

raw cheese, and nibble away to your heart's content. Get back to REAL food and eating like our lean, strong ancestors. And when you do, the weight loss follows.

CHAPTER 2
The Kitchen Cleanout!

Here's a typical list of "food" that the average person trying to lose weight may have on hand. Look in your cabinets and see if any of these fat-fueling foods are lurking in your kitchen:

- Diet shakes—Far from healthy, they're loaded with sugar or high fructose corn syrup, hydrogenated oils, and a lot of synthetic vitamins and additives that add fat to your body, make you hungry, and don't help with weight loss.

- Rice Cakes—Mostly refined starch with little fiber that breaks down immediately into sugar in your body, spiking insulin and promoting fat storage. Did you know that most puffed grains actually have a glycemic value similar to table sugar?

- Protein/Energy bars—Isolated soy protein (virtually unusable by your body), refined grains, hydrogenated oils, tons of sugar, and artificial preservatives. This is a candy bar masquerading as a healthy snack or meal. Don't fall for it.

- Reduced Sugar or Low Fat Desserts—Loaded with artificial sweeteners that are worse for you than sugar, preservatives, and a list of unnatural ingredients about 15 lines long. Nothing at all good in there. A mad scientist's experiment gone awry!

- Diet soda—Sweetened with artificial sweeteners, such as NutraSweet or Splenda, that do more harm than good, raise the insulin levels in your body, cause you to be hungry and store fat. Diet? Think again. This stuff will not help you lose weight—it will make you gain weight!

- Chips, crackers, and cookies—Loaded with hydrogenated (read, "heart attack in a box") fats, highly processed, inflammatory vegetable oils, and processed flours. These high carb foods add fat to your belly almost instantly!

- Refined vegetable oils such as canola oil, corn oil, soybean oil, sunflower oil, safflower oil, or (God forbid!) Crisco. These so-called 'healthy' oils are anything but healthy! These oils are primarily composed of omega 6 fatty acids, which lead to inflammation, heart disease, weight gain and belly flab.

- Breakfast cereal-Advertised as healthy and high fiber; these cereals are made of refined grains and loaded with sugar. They will make you hungrier, spike your blood sugar, and instantly put your body into a fat-storing mode—yes, even the ones that advertise that they help you lose weight. You may as well as eat spoonfuls of sugar.

CHAPTER 3
Grains—What is Wrong With the Food Pyramid?

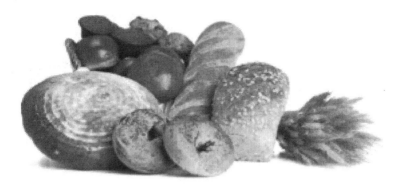

Up until a couple thousand years ago, we humans didn't even eat grains; at least nowhere close to the form we eat today. Grains have been genetically altered to become bigger and contain even more starch than they did in ancient days. Nutrition author Michael Pollan says, in his book, *In Defense of Food*, humans have historically consumed approximately 80,000 different species of edible plants, animals, and fungi.

But here is a shocking and appalling statistic: Currently, the average adult eating a typical modern western diet in countries such as the US, Canada, Australia, etc. consumes approximately 70% of their total caloric intake from only 3 foods—CORN, SOY, AND WHEAT (and that includes all of their derivatives such as corn syrup, corn oil, corn starch, soybean oil, wheat flour, etc).

What is considered a reasonably healthy amount of corn, soy, and wheat in the human diet? Based on tens of thousands of years of human history, and the natural diet of our ancestors (what our digestive systems are genetically programmed to process), this would probably be in the range of about 1% to 5% MAX of our total calories from corn, soy, and wheat.

It's no wonder then that grains are responsible for weight gain, diabetes, inflammation, and degenerative diseases of all kinds. In the 1970's, the average American ate 85 pounds of flour, 84 pounds of sugar, 8 pounds of fried potatoes, and 39 pounds of cooking oil per year. Even then, not so good.

By Mike Geary, Certified Personal Trainer, Certified Nutrition Specialist
& Catherine Ebeling – RN, BSN

Fast forward to the 90's...By 1997, each of us was consuming 122 pounds of flour, 105 pounds of sugar or other sweeteners, 20 pounds of fried potatoes, and 50 pounds of vegetable cooking oils. That's almost a pound of knowingly bad-for-you foods per day! And that doesn't count a whole lot of other junk food, but clearly, this is the reason many are overweight or obese today.

And today, flours are more refined than ever, missing fiber and essential nutrients. The other problem with excess grains in our diet **are anti-nutrients and gluten**, both of which are gut irritants, causing chronic inflammation, digestive issues, nutritional deficiencies, and auto-immune disease in many cases. Processed white flour (alias "enriched wheat flour" or "wheat flour") is missing the two most nutritious and fiber-rich parts of the seed: the outside bran layer and the germ (embryo).

Eating a high starch, grain-based diet will make you feel fatigued, malnourished, constipated, irritable, depressed, and vulnerable to chronic illness. And, refined grain flours fuel high blood sugar levels. High blood sugar leads to insulin release, major fat storage, and increased hunger and cravings. The more grain-based foods a person eats, the more insulin the body produces to manage the fast-digesting carbohydrates. These refined carbohydrates turn to glucose very quickly once in our systems, stimulating the body to produce insulin.

A vicious cycle occurs: the carbs turn to glucose in the body, insulin is released, promoting the storage of fat, making way for rapid weight gain, elevated triglyceride and LDL levels, inflammation, atherosclerosis, type 2 diabetes, and heart disease. Along with all that comes increased hunger and cravings. Excess carbohydrate consumption is like a drug addiction—hard to let go of once you get on that merry-go-round. But this carb/sugar cycle can be deadly in the end, so now is the time to break it.

"Enriched flour," is also very misleading, because only four vitamins and minerals are typically added back, compared to the 15 known nutrients and essential parts of the grain that are removed, along with most of the fiber, some of the antioxidants, and other beneficial substances. Besides the fact that most of these foods are at the top of the list of most frequent food allergies, it's best for anyone to avoid grains, especially wheat and corn for health reasons.

What about Gluten?

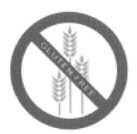 Gluten is a substance that is part of wheat, barley, and rye grains and can often cause stomach upset, bloating, gas, nutritional deficiencies, and inflammation. And if even you do not have full-blown celiac disease, you may still be sensitive to the gluten in grains, as almost a third of the population carries the gene for some degree of gluten sensitivity.

Many people may not even know they may have sensitivity to gluten, but find they feel much better without it. And, the best part is, people often lose weight very quickly as soon as gluten is removed from their diets.

Eating wheat and other grains can cause one to feel lethargic, foggy, groggy, puffy and bloated, and irritable. Many would never connect these symptoms with eating grains, but weight gain, physical, emotional (depression and anxiety are common), and mental symptoms are fairly frequent with gluten sensitivity.

Gluten is the protein portion of wheat, rye and barley. It is so widespread in standard processed food today that it is very hard to escape. Unfortunately, gluten sensitivity is on the rise (notice the "gluten-free" sections at the grocery store?) and it can cause a variety of health problems.

Many grocery stores, health food stores, and restaurants are now offering a big selection of wheat-free/gluten-free foods including breads, pizzas, bagels, cookies, cake mixes, doughnuts, etc. The problem is, gluten-free items are generally made from other refined and heavily processed alternatives such as tapioca starch, potato starch, and corn flour. These processed alternatives are certainly not any healthier!

You are better off avoiding all processed flours altogether! Substituting another refined processed gluten-free grain may bring about a small improvement, but often not the drastic improvement necessary to correct health issues.

The American food supply is also *heavily* based on corn. Bumper crops of corn and government subsidies help to keep corn prices low, which in turn helps to keep many of the junky packaged foods we buy at the store low-priced. Corn and corn by-products are used as fillers, thickeners and sweeteners for just about all processed foods.

Contrary to popular belief, corn is a, not a vegetable, and is really not appropriate as a dietary staple for several reasons: it contains anti-nutrients, excessive omega 6 fats, and creates havoc on blood sugar, when corn products are eaten on a regular basis. Avoid corn in all forms, at all costs!

Corn is not only the most genetically modified grain, but it also contains its own natural toxins and nutrient-blocking ingredients. Corn has a direct effect on blood sugar and insulin and is a key contributor to weight gain. Corn is also a very irritating allergen, and is one of the most common food allergies.

Our bodies cannot exist on such a high quantity of grain-based foods. When archaeologists studied skeletons of Native Americans who ate corn as their primary staple, there was a 50% increase in malnutrition, four times as much incidence of anemia, and three times as much infectious disease. This compared to their more hunter-gatherer ancestors who primarily ate meats and fruits and veggies as opposed to grains.

When civilizations such as the Mayans and Native Americans changed their diet to a corn-based one, these people did not grow as tall, and rates of anemia, arthritis, rickets, and osteoporosis skyrocketed as well. While it is thought that smallpox from the Europeans may be largely responsible for killing off many of these once-strong and invincible warriors, you can't overlook the fact that their diet of corn and grains may have made them much more vulnerable to this deadly illness.

Keep in mind that we are not just talking about corn-on-the-cob (sweet corn) here… we are also talking about most breakfast cereals, chips, and other modern foods promoted by food companies as "healthy". Many of these foods are foods you may not even realize contain corn! There are several reasons researchers have found the health and weight issues caused by a corn-based diet:

- Corn is full of starches and sugars (even though it may not taste sweet) that raise blood sugar and insulin levels, ramping up your appetite and prompting your body to store fat. The starches in corn products are broken down quickly, spiking blood sugar levels, and causing cravings for more carbohydrate-based foods.

- Corn is also a poor source of protein, and deficient in 3 of the 8 essential amino acids: lysine, isoleucine, and tryptophan. The essential amino acids are so-named because they must be obtained from the diet, since the body is unable to manufacture them.

- Corn contains a high amount of phytate, a chemical that binds to iron and inhibits its absorption by the body. Consequently, a diet high in corn and corn by-products will make you more likely to have iron-deficiency anemia and fatigue. Phytate is also a nutrient blocker and inhibits other vitamins and minerals from being absorbed as well.

- Corn is a poor source of certain vitamins and minerals, such as calcium and niacin (B3). Deficiencies of niacin can result in a condition known as Pellagra, which is common in civilizations that eat a lot of corn. Pellagra can cause symptoms like dermatitis, diarrhea, and depression. Since so many of us are corn-eaters, it wouldn't be surprising that this condition is more common than we realize.

- Corn oils are in most processed foods, along with soybean oils. Both corn oil and soybean oil are excessively high in inflammatory omega 6 fats and low in anti-inflammatory omega 3 fats. This throws the delicate balance of omega 6 to omega 3 in your body out of whack, and can cause degenerative diseases and weight gain. In addition, corn oil and soybean oil are highly refined with high heat and solvents, which oxidizes and damages the fragile polyunsaturated fatty acids, and makes them even more inflammatory.

It's not just humans who are eating too much grain. A huge amount of the United States' corn, soy, and wheat crops feed our cattle, because it fattens them up quickly. (Are you beginning to see a connection here?)

Beef from corn and grain-fattened cattle contains much higher ratios of inflammatory omega 6 fatty acids than healthier grass-fed beef which contains more anti-inflammatory omega 3 fats. Most meat that you buy in supermarkets comes from grain-fed animals and not healthy grass-fed animals.

Maximize Your Flat Belly Journey: Get Powerful Fat Loss Secrets From Key Food And Fitness Experts.
http://velocityhousepresents.com/FlatBellyKitchen

Also worth noting, cattle raised on grains actually get something similar to indigestion and acid reflux, (another connection we should pay attention to). This excess acid in their stomachs is exactly what promotes the deadly strain of E. coli O157:H7 to grow and flourish. E.coli O157:H7 is the bacteria responsible for widespread outbreaks of food poisoning and deaths. Grass-fed cattle are far less likely to harbor these toxic bacteria.

My best advice to you is this:

Try at least 2 weeks avoiding all grain products completely. I guarantee you will see drastic improvements in your weight, energy levels, and general outlook! This is easier than you may think...

- For example, instead of having pasta with sauce and meat for dinner, instead have just grass-fed meat, sauce, (try spaghetti squash instead), and veggies topped with Parmesan cheese. It's delicious, filling and does not contain grain.

   Check out some of the healthy grass-fed meats and grass-fed sausages from one of my favorite grass-fed meat sites: www.healthygrassfed.2ya.com

- Another example would be breakfast... instead of cereal, bagels, or muffins, try to base most of your breakfasts on cage-free organic whole eggs with lots of veggies and perhaps some bison sausage or other nitrite-free turkey or chicken sausage.

- If you're very active and need more carbs with your breakfast, instead of grains, a small piece of fruit or some tea with a little bit of raw honey can be great additions to the egg/veggies based breakfast. This delicious and satisfying breakfast keeps blood sugar levels stable, balances your hormones, and eliminates the anti-nutrients found in most grains. Those are just a couple examples, but I think you get the point of how easy this can be.

It may not be realistic for everybody to give up grains completely, so a more realistic plan is to only eat grain based foods (bread, pasta, cereals, etc) on One One of the many other uses of corn is the low-cost sweetener, high-fructose corn syrup. Usage of high-fructose corn syrup has increased by 4,000% since 1973, and the syrup rivals sugar as America's most common sweetener.

The average American now consumes a whopping 40-plus pounds of high-fructose corn syrup each year, according to U. S. Department of Agriculture data. That's an extra 75,281 calories per year per person! And if you look at that in terms of pounds (approx. 3500 calories = 1 pound), you are looking at gaining an extra 22 pounds (of pure fat) their one cheat day each week, and save 6 days per week to be grain-free.

While eliminating refined grains such as corn and wheat can seem a very daunting task, the reward is a return to wonderful health, sparkling eyes, clear skin, clear thinking, and easy weight loss, as your body is again able to get the needed nutrition from the food you eat.
Your body will absolutely thank you!

GRAIN BASED FOODS TO AVOID

- ☐ White, wheat, and rye bread, rolls, buns, muffins
- ☐ Cookies
- ☐ Crackers—Even the ones advertised as "whole grain"
- ☐ Enriched flour pasta
- ☐ Cakes and other desserts
- ☐ Breakfast cereal (Including cereal advertised as "healthy" and "whole grain")
- ☐ Pre-made, packaged gravies, and sauces
- ☐ Packaged macaroni and cheese
- ☐ Instant noodle and soup cups, ramen noodles
- ☐ Packaged dinners with pasta
- ☐ White flour
- ☐ Other types of wheat include: bulgur, durum flour, farina, graham flour, kamut, semolina, and spelt

- ☐ Gluten-free items made with tapioca starch, potato starch, white rice flour and corn flour

- ☐ Corn chips and other tortilla chips; Doritos, Fritos, Sun Chips

- ☐ Corn tortillas

- ☐ Anything with corn, corn starch, maize, or modified food starch as one of the main ingredients

CHAPTER 4
The Evils of Fructose

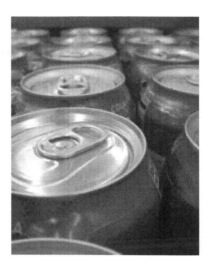

One of the many other uses of corn is the low- cost sweetener, high-fructose corn syrup. Us- age of high-fructose corn syrup has increased by 4,000% since 1973, and the syrup rivals sugar as America's most common sweetener.

The average American now consumes a whopping 40-plus pounds of high-fructose corn syrup each year, according to U. S. De- partment of Agriculture data. That's an extra 75,281 calories per year per person! And if you look at that in terms of pounds (approx. 3500 calories = 1 pound), you are looking at gaining an extra 22 pounds (of pure fat) a year. Most of that comes from soda, energy drinks, and juice (even 100% fruit juice) drinks.

Teenagers typically get 15 to 20 teaspoons per day of added sugars from high-fructose corn syrup—just from drinking soft drinks! Another study shows that soft drinks have replaced milk as a dietary staple and have become the third-most-common breakfast food.

Starting the day with a sugar high leads to a crash in about 2 hours and causes more hunger and weight gain. No wonder so many teens are overweight! If the average American could cut just *one* soft drink, juice, or sugared water drink a *day* they would immediately lose 10 pounds a year!

Since 2009, approximately 25% of the average American's caloric intake comes from sugars—mostly high fructose corn syrup! That's 25% of the diet filled with not only empty, but also harmful calories! The next time you're at the supermarket, pick up any several different bottled drinks—including juice, energy or sport drinks—and check out the ingredients label. Generally the first or second ingredient will be high fructose corn syrup or HFCS.

Now, go through the rest of the grocery store and read the ingredients of random items that you may not think contain sugar—like ketchup, salad dressing, spaghetti sauce, soups, cereals, and marinades. You will probably see corn syrup in most everything. HFCS is everywhere! It is entirely possible that 80% of the processed food you consume is chock–full of HFCS. When you see how easily high fructose corn syrup is stored as fat, it's no wonder there is so much obesity, heart disease, and diabetes.

What is high fructose corn syrup? High fructose corn syrup not a natural product like the corn producers would like us to believe, but a chemically altered substance, far different than just regular corn syrup. That chemical alteration changes corn syrup from a compound that is mainly glucose (a simple sugar which our bodies easily handle) to around 50% fructose (though some can range as high as 90% fructose) with the remainder being glucose and other sugars.

A study in 2004 reported in the American Journal of Clinical Nutrition cites the increase in consumption of HFCS to be 4000% between 1970 and 1990! (While consumption of high fructose corn syrup has actually decreased slightly in the past year or so, sugar consumption is up 10%). This is way higher than any other increase of any other food or food group. Too bad we haven't increased our intake of fruits and vegetables by that amount—our country would be in far better health—and much slimmer!

Fructose is converted to fat in the body more easily than any other sugar.

How does this work? Unlike glucose, fructose is metabolized 100% in the liver. Fructose turns into triglycerides (fats), and LDL cholesterol. (Yes, it's true—fructose is far worse for your heart and cholesterol levels than butter, eggs, and steak!)

Because fructose is a sugar, it stimulates the body to secrete insulin. Insulin triggers the body to store fat. Well since the fructose has very efficiently been turned into fatty acids, they are almost instantly stored in the cells as fat. The rest of those fat particles are stored in the liver or the muscles, which can lead to something called "non-alcoholic fatty liver disease," or NAFLD.

While the liver is metabolizing the fructose into fats, it also creates metabolic by-products such as uric acid. Uric acid is known for being a primary cause of gout, a very painful form of arthritis. Uric acid can also contribute to high blood pressure. The negative effects of excess fructose also include increased risk of heart attacks, pancreatitis, obesity, fatty liver disease, and insulin resistance, as well as all the diseases that are associated with type 2 diabetes and obesity.

Fructose actually promotes overeating. Don't let anyone tell you that "sugar is just sugar." There are major differences in the type of sugar you eat, and how your body processes it. Fructose leads directly to increased belly fat and disease—no question about it. But beware of regular table sugar—it is made up of about 40% fructose as well, and can be almost just as harmful as corn syrup.

High fructose corn syrup almost always comes from genetically modified corn, which is full of its own problems and health concerns. In studies done on animals, scientist found that animals fed genetically modified corn developed serious, and often deadly health issues in the digestive system, reproductive system, blood, kidneys and liver.

High-fructose corn syrup (HFCS) often contains mercury as well. Mercury acts as a toxin to your brain and nervous system, and is especially dangerous for pregnant women and small children. Even in low doses, mercury can interfere with brain development, memory and learning ability.

Mercury poisoning in adults is a serious risk as well, and has been linked to Alzheimer's, dementia, fertility problems, memory, and vision loss. It can also cause extreme fatigue and neuromuscular dysfunction. Other studies show that mercury causes psychological, neurological, and immunological problems.

Although the makers of HFCS like to claim that it's natural, HFCS is a highly refined product that would *never* exist in nature. Converting corn to HFCS is a very extensive process, and mercury is used in the production of the HFCS.

You CAN avoid high fructose corn syrup if you make a concerted effort to focus your diet on whole, healthy, natural foods. If you do purchase processed foods, make sure you read the label ... and put it back on the shelf if it lists high-fructose corn syrup, sugar, or dextrose (a sugar derived from corn), as one of the first or second ingredients.

Food companies are starting to notice that consumers are avoiding high fructose corn syrup, and many are beginning to use regular sugar again. Some companies are even beginning to use the natural (better for you) low-calorie sweetener, stevia.

GETTING RID OF FRUCTOSE

☐ Any kind of soda (Coke, Pepsi, 7-up, Dr. Pepper, etc.)

☐ Flavored drinks or juices, even 100% real fruit juice

☐ Lemonade

☐ Sweetened sports drinks.

☐ Applesauce, fruit cocktail, canned fruits

☐ Barbeque sauces, marinades, ketchup, spaghetti sauce, steak sauce

☐ Alcoholic drink mixes (like margarita mix, etc)

☐ Puddings, Jell-O, flavored yogurt

☐ Ice cream products, frozen yogurt

☐ Premade cakes, desserts

☐ Kid's juice box drinks

☐ Candy

☐ Cereals

- Any kind of syrup other than pure 100% maple syrup

- Granola bars

- Anything pre-made and pre-packaged most likely has corn syrup or HFCS in it

Maximize Your Flat Belly Journey: Get Powerful Fat Loss Secrets From Key Food And Fitness Experts.
http://velocityhousepresents.com/FlatBellyKitchen

CHAPTER 5
The Bad Fats—You May be Shocked!

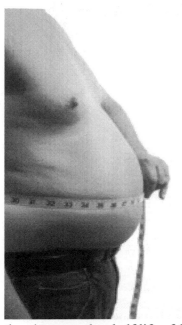

We have all been told we should avoid saturated fat. But the fact is, the right fats will actually make you leaner. Eating the wrong kinds of fat will not only make you fat, but contribute to a variety of other diseases and health issues, as well as premature aging. And contrary to popular belief, unhealthy fats are mostly trans fats and vegetable oils—not saturated fats like butter, lard or coconut oil.

Trans fats are finally starting to be noticed for being extremely unhealthy. Trans fats are not natural fats. They are vegetable oils artificially transformed with hydrogen under high heat, pressure, and chemicals. This makes an oil turn into something more like a solid at room temperature. Food manufacturers have been using trans fats because they increase the shelf life of foods, but these fats have no benefits in our bodies and in fact are highly destructive.

Trans fats actually affect your cell membranes (which are made of lipids) and cause them to become brittle and unable to properly metabolize nutrients and calories. Think about that internal damage next time you consider eating those French fries, donuts, or fried chicken, and you may change your mind.

A healthy cell has a living, breathing membrane made of fatty acids that transmits and utilizes nutrients properly. When you think of a cell affected by trans fats, think of a cell with a hard shell around it, instead of a breathing membrane. That hard shell actually smothers the cell, and causes it to become dysfunctional, blocking proper metabolism, nutrition, and creating an inability to respond to glucose. Inflammation in the body increases. This not only leads to diseases like diabetes and heart disease, but also weight gain, and an inability to fight infections and cancers.

In spite of the dangers of trans fats, they are still found in many processed and baked foods: cookies, crackers, cake icing, snack chips, stick margarine, and microwave popcorn to name just a few. Most of the trans fat in the modern diet comes from commercially produced hydrogenated vegetable oil.

Margarine—and other substitute-butter spreads—Crisco, and other solid short-enings are examples of trans fats. Butter is far better to eat than these artificial unhealthy substitutes. In fact, butter can actually be healthy, especially if it's grass-fed organic butter. I have an article on my blog about how real grass-fed butter can actually HELP you to lose fat.

What about vegetable oils? Isn't vegetable oil supposed to be a healthy alternative to saturated fats like butter and lard? Keep in mind that one of the reasons they are touted as "healthy" has to do with how cheap vegetable oils are to produce, and the heavy marketing budgets behind the companies that push vegetable oils.

Oils like canola, corn, soybean, and sunflower have been pushed as the healthy substitutes for saturated fats. Sunflower oil, soy oil, corn oil, and canola oils still seem to be popular choices for cooking. However, research has painted a very different picture. These vegetable oils that are primarily made up of omega 6 fatty acids, contribute to inflammation in the body and upset the ratio of omega 3 fatty acids to omega 6 fatty acids. Omega 3 fatty acids are the healthy fatty acids found in the fat of wild caught fish and grass-fed meats.

While we do need some omega 6 fatty acids in our diet, we get far too much in our diet, compared to omega 3 fats. Excess consumption of omega 6 oils leads to increased health problems including inflammatory diseases like auto-immune diseases and cardiovascular disease.

The fats in our diet changed drastically in the early 1900's, when margarine, made of refined vegetable oil, began being consumed. We were told it was a healthier choice. At the same time, our consumption of omega 3 fatty acids from foods such as wild caught fish, grass-fed beef, wild game, and green, leafy vegetables decreased. Our early ancestors ate about a 1:1 ratio of omega 6 fats to omega 3 fats. Unfortunately, this ratio is now about 20 to 1 in North America (and most modernized diets around the world) today. In other words, we are eating 20 times as much omega 6 fats compared to omega 3 fats.

Maximize Your Flat Belly Journey: Get Powerful Fat Loss Secrets From Key Food And Fitness Experts.
http://velocityhousepresents.com/FlatBellyKitchen

By Mike Geary, Certified Personal Trainer, Certified Nutrition Specialist
& Catherine Ebeling – RN, BSN

Vegetable oils, in spite of the fact that we have been told they are healthy, are actually quite damaging to the body, causing increases in the rates of lung and reproductive cancers. Diets high in vegetable oils–especially hydrogenated vegetable oils, can cause irritability, learning disabilities, liver toxicity, decreased immune function, mental and physical problems in growing children, increased uric acid, abnormal fatty acid profiles, dementia, and chromosomal damage because they accelerate aging.

Vegetable oils also stimulate the production of prostaglandins (inflammatory chemicals in the body) leading to a variety of health issues ranging from arthritis and other autoimmune diseases, and even PMS. This inflammation irritates blood vessels, setting the stage for cholesterol deposits and blood clots, causing heart attacks and strokes.

Sad to say, cholesterol in the diet has been wrongly accused of being the culprit behind heart disease, because it is much more likely that the omega 6 fats (as well as trans fats, sugars, and other inflammatory foods in the average diet) that are behind this health problem. A 1994 study from a leading medical journal showed that almost three quarters of the fat in clogged arteries are from vegetable oils, not saturated fats. The "artery clogging" fats are more likely to be caused by vegetable oils, not animal fat!

Vegetable oils also become toxic when heated. High heat alters the structure of the oils making them even more damaging to your body! And heating vegetable oils over and over again increases the toxicity even more. Think of that the next time you eat an order of fast food French fries!

On a side note, this is one little trick that I've used over the years to train myself to actually be repulsed by French fries (even though I used to love them years ago). I've studied the biochemistry of what happens to oil, used in a deep fryer, which is usually hydrogenated, and also heated and reheated many times. Once it has been used repeatedly, the oils begin to react as almost a poison inside your body. This actually makes it easy to view deep fried food like French fries as repulsive instead of something to crave.

Also interesting is a study done by a plastic surgeon found that people who consumed lots of vegetable oils had far more facial wrinkles than those who used traditional animal fats. So you see, these once so-called healthy oils are aging the body. Even the doctors and researchers who promoted the use of omega 6 vegetable oils as part of a healthy diet are now aware of their dangers. Scientists have actually warned against including too many polyunsaturated vegetable oils in the diet for several years.

Examples of bad for you vegetable oils are: canola oil, soybean oil, sunflower oil, corn oil, and safflower oil. All these oils are highly processed and unhealthy. If you are going to use any type of vegetable oils, extra virgin olive is good, as long as you are not using heat with it. Any vegetable oil that is cold processed is healthier for you, again, though as long as you are not using it to cook with high heat. For cooking, use coconut oil. It is much better for you, and heating it does not harm it.

Totally avoid anything that lists as an ingredient, "partially hydrogenated" or "hydrogenated_____"! And remember that even canola oil, although it's often promoted as "healthy," is truly not good for you. I previously wrote a thorough article on that topic on my site, and you can read the full story of why canola oil is bad for you here.

One of the most important things you can do for your health, prevention of disease, and for your waistline, is to try to avoid omega 6 oils and fats, and to strive to include more foods that are high in omega 3 fats. As I said earlier, it's best to eat approximately a 2:1 ratio of omega fats (although the average American has a terrible 20:1 ratio).

High quality fish oil, or even the more potent Krill oil, can really help your intake of omega 3 fats. In addition, Krill oil has the added benefits of having higher absorption due to the phospholipids contained, as well as the powerful antioxidant, astaxanthin, which gives krill oil up to 47x more antioxidant power than fish oil. With that said, there are powerful benefits to both fish oil and krill oil, and one benefit of fish oil is simply higher doses of omega 3's and DHA/EPA.

BAD FATS TO AVOID

☐ Vegetable oils—cottonseed oil, soybean oil, corn oil, canola oil, sunflower oil, safflower oil

31

☐ Any oil that starts out with "partially hydrogenated" or "hydrogenated"

☐ Margarine of any kind or any kind of "healthy" butter substitute or spread

☐ Baked goods like cookies, snack cakes, or doughnuts with hydrogenated fats

☐ Microwave popcorn, especially the ones with "butter" flavoring

☐ Crisco

☐ Frozen foods like French fries, tater tots, snack foods, TV dinners

☐ Some peanut butters (natural peanut butters don't have added trans fats but many other brands do have "partially hydrogenated" oils)

☐ Cake icing, especially decorated cakes

☐ Frozen breaded prepared meats like chicken tenders, etc.

☐ Some whipped toppings

☐ Non dairy coffee creamers (real organic cream or coconut milk is healthier)

☐ Fast food milk shakes

☐ Deep fried foods, especially from restaurants – fries, fried chicken, fried fish, etc.

☐ Velveeta cheese or other processed packaged (squirt can) cheese

CHAPTER 6
Artificial Sweeteners—Good or Bad?

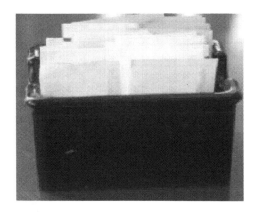

Do diet sweeteners really help you lose weight, or do you eat more and gain weight in the long run? Could it be that diet sweeteners can make you fat? The fact is, diet sweeteners can actually make you gain weight, because they trick your body and don't feed it what it actually needs.

According to researchers, there is no actual evidence that sugar substitutes help people lose weight. These days, more and more data suggests that these chemical sweeteners may actually stimulate your appetite and insulin response.

Anyone who cares about their health should stay away from the highly toxic sweetener aspartame (NutraSweet) and other questionable sweeteners such as sucralose (Splenda), saccharin (Sweet-n-Low), and acesulfame-k.

Artificial sweeteners are chemical concoctions that you should not eat. They have absolutely NO food value, they trick the body into thinking it is eating something sweet, and they contain by-products of harmful toxins.

How do artificial sweeteners fool the body? Aspartame, for instance, doesn't have any calories, but one of its ingredients, the amino acid phenylalanine, blocks the production of serotonin, a natural brain chemical that, among other things, controls food cravings.

When you have a shortage of serotonin in the brain, it will make your brain and body crave the foods that help make more serotonin—and those happen to be the starchy, high-calorie, carbohydrate-rich snacks that can totally sabotage a diet. As you increase the amount of aspartame you take in, the more intense your cravings for these foods will be.

This leads to a vicious cycle of cravings, eating, eating more artificial sweeteners, and more cravings. Long term, you are looking at weight gain as the primary result. Artificial sweeteners as diet food? Hardly! Scientists now suspect that something additional is going on in many people who have been using artificial sweeteners. The sweet taste of no-calorie sweeteners triggers an insulin release, even when there is no food intake to feed the cells.

Normally, when we eat sugars, they are broken down into glucose, the form of sugar our body uses, which then enters the blood stream. Insulin, (secreted by the pancreas) unlocks the cells and allows blood sugar into our cells to supply energy and maintain normal blood sugar levels.

The problem is, an insulin-sensitive person who uses artificial sweeteners confuses their body into thinking food has been eaten, so insulin is released. When insulin is released, it lowers your blood sugar, but it also triggers your appetite.

As soon as your body discovers it there is no food in your system, it creates strong cravings that will only stop by eating food that raises the blood sugar. It becomes hard to avoid high-calorie sugary snacks at this point, and you get into a cycle of hunger, cravings and snacks.

Six artificial sweeteners have been approved by the FDA. In addition to saccharin (Sweet-n-Low), sucralose (Splenda) and aspartame (NutraSweet), there is acesulfame potassium, also called Ace-K and marketed as Sunett and Sweet One, and Neotame. More recently, a natural (non-artificial) sweetener derived from the stevia plant is being used in some packaged foods and drinks. The sweetener is called stevia and is being marketed under several names such as Truvia (an extracted portion of the stevia herb), or just pure stevia in many brands.

Saccharin was the first of the artificial sweetener on the market. Saccharin has no calories and is hundreds of times sweeter than sugar. Many people notice an unpleasant bitter aftertaste in foods sweetened with this product. Saccharin has been a long-standing sugar substitute, with many faithful followers, but it has had issues related to health from the time it came out on the market. Saccharin is a synthetic, white crystalline powder with no nutritional value, and the body has a hard time digesting it. Saccharin is still the third most popular artificial sweetener, after sucralose and aspartame.

Do you know how saccharin was discovered? You may be surprised. Maybe this knowledge will help you decide on whether or not to include it in your diet! In 1879, a chemist discovered this sweetener (also known as benzoic sulfinide or E954) when he was researching coal tar derivatives. The chemist was not trying to discover a new sweetener, or a food product at all. It was purely by accident that he discovered his new product tasted sweet. How did he find out? Who knows? Maybe he accidentally touched his mouth while working. Probably not a great thing to do—tasting chemicals, but he did.

After discovering its sweetness, it was marketed as a sweetener, and controversy over the safety of this artificial sweetener has followed along ever since. In 1977, it was thought that saccharin caused cancer, after a study connected it to bladder tumors in mice. The US National Toxicology Program then put saccharin on its cancer causing list—officially declaring it a human carcinogen. Cyclamate, an earlier version of the sweetener, had been banned in 1970 for similar reasons. The U.S. Food and Drug Administration decided that saccharin should carry a warning label regarding its cancer connection.

The warning label has since been removed due to inconclusive evidence of the saccharin and cancer connection in humans, but it is still a sweetener to be treated with caution and it is certainly not healthy in the long run. Saccharin can cause reactions like these in some sensitive people:

- Itching
- Hives
- Eczema
- Nausea
- Headaches
- Diarrhea
- Excessive urination
- Wheezing
- Tongue blisters

Next time you reach for that pink package to sweeten your coffee or tea, remember you are adding a coal tar derivative. Does that sound good for your health?

Aspartame has been on the market for over twenty years, and although there have been many health concerns associated with this artificial sweetener, it still remains a staple of the no-calorie artificial sweeteners, and is still marketed in many products.

Aside from the weight gain problems, there are also large portions of the population who suffer from unhealthy side effects associated with aspartame. Individuals who do not have immediate reactions may still be susceptible to the long-term damage caused by the excitatory amino acids contained in aspartame: phenylalanine, methanol, and DKP.

Adverse reactions and side effects of aspartame include:

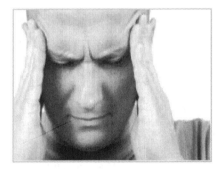

• Vision problems
• Tinnitus—ringing or buzzing sounds
• Noise sensitivity or hearing impairment
• Epileptic seizures
• Headaches, migraines, dizziness
• Depression
• Irritability
• Aggression
• Anxiety
• Palpitations, tachycardia
• Stomach and abdominal pain
• Itching
• Rashes, hives

While Splenda (sucralose) seems to be safer than aspartame (NutraSweet, Equal) there still has not been enough convincing evidence to prove Splenda's safety, and generally should be considered unsafe to use as a low-calorie sweetener.

Splenda claims to be 'made from sugar,' and 'natural,' because it is made partially from sucrose, which is a natural sugar. But sucralose is NOT at all natural; it is a chemically created synthetic compound, modified by adding chlorine atoms to sugar.

Unfortunately, this covalently bonded chlorine is like ingesting small amounts of chlorinated pesticides. And coincidentally, sucralose was actually discovered in the 1970's by scientists who were trying to create a new pesticide! Since a no-calorie sweetener is much more marketable than a pesticide, it was named "Splenda" and advertised as a 'natural' substitute for sugar. Little does the public know that this sweetener was once almost bug-killer. If it kills bugs, it seems very likely that it is harmful to humans as well. Do you really want to be sweetening your food or drinks with pesticides?

How does Splenda work? Most of it passes through the body without being digested, however, people with healthy GI tracts end up absorbing more of the Splenda, and that means more chlorine is absorbed into the body, along with the resulting health hazards. Even the research done by Splenda's own manufacturers is scary. Studies revealed that test animals suffered from nasty side effects such as enlarged livers and kidneys, and shrunken thymus glands, and these were only the short-term studies. What happens long-term?

Splenda was rushed to the marketplace before any long-term studies were completed. If Splenda is dangerous in smaller doses, but what about larger amounts of Splenda and the chlorine it contains? The problem with that is that many of the sugar-free, and low-calorie diet foods now use Splenda in their recipes. People on sugar-free and low calorie diets are eating this product several times a day in different foods and drinks.

Many people can actually be allergic to sucralose, and the reactions can be everything from rashes, panic attacks, headaches, to intestinal cramping, diarrhea, muscle aches, and stomach pain. Allergic reactions may not show up the first time, but may suddenly appear after several exposures.

There is also evidence that sucralose can damage the healthy probiotic colonies living in your gut, and this can harm both digestion and your immune system. While we don't know if sucralose is as toxic as aspartame, it is clear that years and years of use may contribute to serious immunological and neurological disorders.

Maximize Your Flat Belly Journey: Get Powerful Fat Loss Secrets From Key Food And Fitness Experts.
http://velocityhousepresents.com/FlatBellyKitchen

According to Dr. Joseph Mercola (www.mercola.com), the following symptoms were observed within 24-hours of eating Splenda products:

- Redness, itching, swelling, blistering, weeping, crusting, rash, eruptions, or hives. This is the most common allergic symptom that people have.

- Wheezing, tightness, cough, or shortness of breath.

- Swelling of the face, eyelids, lips, tongue, or throat.

- Headaches and migraines.

- Stuffy nose, runny nose, sneezing.

- Red, itchy, swollen, or watery eyes.

- Bloating, gas, pain, nausea, vomiting, diarrhea, or bloody diarrhea.

- Heart palpitations or fluttering.

- Joint pains or aches.

- Anxiety, dizziness, spaced-out sensation, depression.

There are many other natural sweeteners that are much healthier choices and do not contain a list of frightening side effects when ingested. I will cover these healthy options in depth later in this book. My preferred natural sweeteners are stevia (when wanting to reduce sugar calories), or raw honey and 100% organic maple syrup (both of which do contain sugar, but also contain beneficial nutrients.

SUGAR FREE FOODS TO AVOID

- ☐ Diet Sodas
- ☐ Crystal Lite Drink Mixes
- ☐ Sugar Free Kool-Aid
- ☐ Sugar Free Drinks of all Kinds
- ☐ Sugar Free Sports Drinks

- ☐ Sugar Free Yogurt

- ☐ Sugar Free Snacks and Desserts

- ☐ Sugar Free Ice Cream

- ☐ Sugar Free Syrups, Jams, and Jellies

- ☐ Sugar Free Gum

- ☐ Sugar Free Candy

- ☐ Many protein powders, protein shakes, and bars also contain artificial sweeteners in heavy doses, so read labels!

- ☐ Anything that says "Sugar Free" read the label; most likely it contains one of the artificial sweeteners mentioned.

Maximize Your Flat Belly Journey: Get Powerful Fat Loss Secrets From Key Food And Fitness Experts.
http://velocityhousepresents.com/FlatBellyKitchen

CHAPTER 7
Dairy—Does it Do a Body Good?

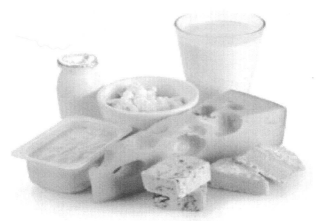

Although milk is promoted as a healthy food, there are many problems with commercial pasteurized dairy products. There is only <u>one</u> form of healthy milk, and that is raw (unpasteurized, unhomogenized) milk from grass-fed healthy cows. Unfortunately, virtually all of the milk sold in stores in the US has been pasteurized and homogenized (and is almost always from corn-fed feedlot cows), thus turning a healthy food into an unhealthy one. While the dairy industry promotes pasteurized milk as being wholesome and healthy, it is not.

You may be surprised to know that studies show commercial, pasteurized milk may play a role in a variety of health problems, including: diabetes, prostate cancer, rheumatoid arthritis, atherosclerosis, anemia, MS, leukemia and ovarian cancer. If you are willing to look, you would find that that there are many reports and studies on pasteurized milk, and most of them are not favorable.

Some of the health problems associated with milk include: intestinal irritation and bleeding, anemia, allergic reactions, sinusitis, heart disease, arthritis, leukemia, lymphoma, cancer. Health problems in children can include bedwetting, colic, childhood diabetes, ear infections, and asthma. Then there is the issue of milk contaminated with blood and white blood cells (pus), as well as chemicals, drugs and insecticides. How healthy and wholesome does milk sound now?

One of the biggest problems with conventional milk is the way dairy cows are raised. Fifty years ago, a dairy cow normally produced about 2,000 pounds of milk a year. Today, in a commercialized dairy setting, dairy cows produce closer to 50,000 pounds of milk. This is certainly not natural! Dairy cows are given various drugs, growth hormones, antibiotics, and forcefed to accomplish this.

Cows now receive Bovine Growth Hormone (BGH) as well to stimulate milk production. The problem with all of this is that the drugs, hormones, chemicals and toxins the dairy cows are exposed to come out in the milk. So, it seems we aren't really drinking wholesome, pure milk after all!

Research on BGH shows that it seems to stimulate the growth of cancerous tumors. It makes perfect sense that if this unnatural drug can stimulate growth, then it can stimulate the growth of cancer as well. It is also thought to increase breast cancer rates in women as well. Many countries have already banned BGH because of safety concerns. Because BGH dramatically increases the cow's milk supply, it also causes a huge increase (50 to 70 %) in mastitis (udder infections) in dairy cows. This infection requires antibiotics, and the leftover antibiotics then appear in the milk we drink.

Because of the mastitis, there are white blood cells in the milk from infections. If you don't already know this, I'm sorry to tell you, but white cells are otherwise known as 'pus.' A-not-too-appetizing fact is that the USDA allows commercially produced milk to contain from one to one and a half million white blood cells per milliliter.

Over 50% of all the antibiotics produced in this country for both humans and animals go directly into animal feed! Ideally, antibiotics should be used in farming only when necessary to treat infections. But commercial dairy cows are raised in poor, dirty conditions, and they are not healthy animals. So they are fed a constant supply of antibiotics from birth until death.

That means we are exposed to more antibiotics than we realize, just by drinking commercial milk. Commercial milk actually contains traces of up to 80 different antibiotics!

Side note: *If you had not already heard the news, there is scientific evidence* *that antibiotics use in humans can actually increase your abdominal fat due to the disruption of proper balance in your gut flora. Read that article if you're interested in more on that topic.*

Pure, wholesome milk? Yuck! It is more like a disgusting cocktail of antibiotics, chemicals, hormones and pus. Commercial pasteurized milk is not a health food and should be avoided at all costs. Milk is empty calories that just add pounds to your body, and fills you with chemicals.

But wait, there's more! Pasteurization further degrades milk and makes it even unhealthier. Since dairy cattle are raised on grain, not grass, this totally changes the composition of the fats in milk, especially the very important and healthy fatty acids—omega 3's and CLA.

Pasteurizing milk actually began in the 1920's to kill pathogens that got into the milk that caused tuberculosis, infant diarrhea, intestinal dysentery, and other diseases caused by poor animal nutrition and dirty production methods. According to Sally Fallon of the Weston Price Foundation:

> *"Heat alters milk's amino acids, lysine and tyrosine, making the whole complex of proteins less available; it promotes rancidity of unsaturated fatty acids and destruction of vitamins. Vitamin C loss in pasteurization usually exceeds 50 percent; loss of other water-soluble vitamins can run as high as 80 percent. Pasteurization alters milk's mineral components such as calcium, chlorine, magnesium, phosphorus, potassium, sodium and sulphur as well as many trace minerals, making them less available. There is some evidence that pasteurization alters lactose, making it more readily absorbable."*

When milk is heat pasteurized, the protein molecules actually change shape and composition, making them much harder for our bodies to break down and digest. A simple protein molecule becomes a tightly folded molecule. This milk then puts an unnecessary strain on our digestive system to produce digestive enzymes to break this down. Many people's bodies are simply incapable of breaking this complex protein down.

This is partly the reason why milk consumption has been linked with diabetes.

It is a strain on the pancreas to produce enzymes. It is also the reason behind many milk allergies. It is the protein portion— the casein— that becomes difficult to digest after pasteurization, thus causing many autoimmune and allergic reactions.

In the elderly, and those with milk intolerance or other digestive disorders, milk passes through the intestinal walls not fully digested. These large particles can clog the absorbent areas of the small intestine, which then prevents vital nutrients from getting in. The result is allergies, chronic fatigue, lowered immune response, and a variety of other degenerative diseases.

Because the milk is heated in pasteurization, the heat also destroys the active, healthy enzymes in milk–in fact, the test for successful pasteurization is absence of enzymes. These enzymes are especially important to help our body break down and use all the healthy nutrients in milk, including calcium. This is one of the reasons people with osteoporosis cannot get calcium from pasteurized milk. The same goes for the healthy fats milk contains. Lipase is one of the enzymes in raw milk that helps the body digest the butterfat that contains conjugated linoleic acid (CLA) and Omega 3 fats—both extremely healthy to the body in their cancer-fighting and heart-healthy abilities (as well as helping with fat burning and muscle building).

Last but not least, chemicals are often added after pasteurization to suppress the odor and restore some of the taste. Then it is homogenized to keep the fat from separating. Homogenization breaks up the healthy fat particles into microscopic particles and distributes the fat throughout the milk. This process unnaturally exposes the fat to more air, oxidizing the fat, and increasing the chances of spoiling. Because homogenized milk contains oxidized fats, it has been linked to heart disease and atherosclerosis.

When you look at production process of commercial milk, it should be no surprise that so many people are either lactose intolerant or allergic to milk. Allergic reactions can cause symptoms like diarrhea, vomiting (even projectile vomiting), stomach pain, depression, cramping, gas, bloating, nausea, headaches, asthma, eczema, sinus and chest congestion, earaches, severe acne, and sore throat.

Commercial milk consumption is linked to other health conditions as well,

such as asthma, atherosclerosis, diabetes and juvenile diabetes, chronic infections (especially upper respiratory and ear infections), obesity, osteoporosis
and prostate, ovarian, breast, and colon cancer. Did you know that a calf fed
pasteurized milk will die before it matures? How then, can you believe that
there is anything good about pasteurized, processed, homogenized milk?

Why add the empty calories, toxins, antibiotics and growth hormones? Raw,
unpasteurized, un-homogenized milk from healthy grass-fed cows is actually
the best source of milk to drink. Milk can be one of the healthiest foods available in its raw and unprocessed state. See more about raw milk in Part 2 of
this book.

MILK PRODUCTS TO AVOID

☐ Pasteurized milk—especially skim milk, or 2% milk. Organic milk is better
but it is still pasteurized and homogenized.

☐ Pasteurized cottage cheese

☐ Pasteurized yogurt—especially the kind with fruit and sugar

☐ Pasteurized sour cream

☐ Pasteurized, processed cheese

☐ Pasteurized chocolate milk

☐ Pasteurized cream

☐ Frozen yogurt—especially 'low fat' frozen yogurt

☐ Any pasteurized processed dairy product. Hint: because of laws regarding
raw dairy in the US, you cannot purchase anything but pasteurized milk in a
grocery store. You can however, buy raw cheese at most stores.

CHAPTER 8
To Eat or Not to Eat—Meat, Fish, or Poultry

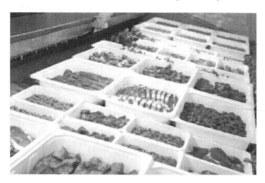

Not all meat you buy is the same. In fact, there is a world of difference, depending on how it is raised. Commercial meat production has sadly changed a healthy lean protein, into an industrialized factory food full of toxins, which is now a health hazard. Animals raised for conventional meat in most grocery stores are raised and slaughtered under inhumane cruel conditions, and fed an unhealthy, unnatural diet that makes them sick and diseased. But read on, because there ARE healthy meats that you can choose!

Since the 1980's, big mergers have resulted in concentrating 80% of the beef industry in the U.S. under the control of four huge corporations. What used to be idyllic country farms with contented grazing cattle has turned into huge industrialized factory farms of dirty, disgusting feedlots.

Most beef cattle start out on a range, eating grass, but upon reaching maturity, they are transported to a feedlot to be fattened up on a diet of grain, and readied for slaughter. They spend their last 3-4 months at feedlots, crowded by the thousands into dirty, manure-laden pens. The air is thick with dangerous bacteria, infectious disease, dust and fecal matter, putting the cattle at risk for respiratory disease and a host of other diseases. Eventually, all of them will wind up at the slaughterhouse.

Feedlot cattle are injected regularly with growth hormones and antibiotics. Because they are fed grain and other food by-products to fatten them up very quickly and profitably, the cattle often have upset digestive systems and they become even sicker and unhealthier in general. Cattle eating grain develop overly acidic stomachs (much like heartburn and acid reflux humans get), which become a breeding ground for the very dangerous form of E.coli bacteria, which can sicken and kill humans.

Grains (often contaminated with fungus and fungicides) are used to fatten up livestock at the expense of their natural diet of green grass and hay. The main ingredients are genetically modified corn and soy. To further cut costs, the feed may also contain "by-product feedstuff" such as municipal garbage, stale pastry, chicken feathers, gum and stale candy.

In the U.S. alone, farmers add around 10 million pounds of antibiotics into the food and water supply of livestock. These antibiotics are not intended to fight or prevent disease, but actually used to fatten up the livestock, which is one of the side effects of the antibiotics. All of the antibiotics in the meat you are eating can lead to antibiotic resistance in your body. And, if these antibiotics work to fatten cattle, guess what they can do to your body?

Cattle are transported several times during their short lifetimes, and they may have to travel hundreds or thousands of miles during a single trip. Long journeys are very stressful to the cattle, and contribute to even more disease and death.

A standard beef slaughterhouse kills about 250 cattle an hour. The high speed of the processing makes it difficult to treat animals humanely. According to a meat and poultry industry article, "Good handling is extremely difficult if equipment is 'maxed out' all the time. It is impossible to have a good attitude towards the cattle if the employees are stressed and constantly rushed, always trying to increase production in as little time as possible."

Nearly all the meat, eggs, and dairy products that you find in the supermarket come from animals raised in large facilities called CAFOs or "Confined Animal Feeding Operations." These highly mechanized operations provide a year-round supply of food at a reasonable price. Although the meat is cheap and convenient, factory farming is creating a variety of problems, including:

- Animal disease, abuse, and inhumane treatment
- Air, land, and water pollution
- The unnecessary use of hormones, antibiotics, and other drugs which end up in the meat you are eating
- Unhealthy fats that cause inflammation and heart disease
- Food with decreased nutritional value

What about those dangerous saturated fats you ask? Well, it is becoming more widely known that saturated fat per se is NOT the real culprit in heart disease and other degenerative diseases. Read this article link below for more details: http://www.truthaboutabs.com/saturated-fat-is-not-evil.html

The fat in a grain-fed cow is not healthy. Grain fed beef contains high amounts of inflammatory (hence, artery clogging) omega 6 fatty acids. One reason Americans are so unhealthy and have a lot of inflammation in their bodies is due to excessively high amounts of processed omega 6 fatty acids in our diets in relation to omega 3 fatty acids.

According to the Journal of Animal Science, grain fed beef or bison can have an omega 6 to omega 3 ratio higher than 20:1. On the other hand, grass-fed beef or bison typically contains a much healthier omega 6 to omega 3 ratio of between 2:1 to 4:1, and about 5 times as much CLA (a healthy fat that helps support fat burning and muscle building).

When this recommended ratio of 2:1 to 3:1 omega 6 to omega 3 fats is exceeded, health problems begin to emerge due to an unhealthy imbalance. Excess omega 6 fatty acids contribute to inflammation in our bodies, and in our arteries, which is the starting point for arterial plaque buildup.

Animals raised on their natural diet of grass have high levels of nutrients such as Conjugated Linoleic Acid (CLA), omega 3 fats, healthy proteins, vitamins, minerals and digestive enzymes. But even a small amount of grain feeding can change the nutrition in the meat. Just 30 days on a grain-based diet can ruin 200 days of grass-grazing benefits.

By Mike Geary, Certified Personal Trainer, Certified Nutrition Specialist
& Catherine Ebeling – RN, BSN

On top of all that, growth hormones given for quick weight gain don't create healthy, lean muscle. Grain fed cattle don't get to walk around and graze like their pasture-raised, grass-fed counterparts, so the grain fed cattle develop fatty, marbled muscle, which is the hallmark of their high carbohydrate diet. This phenomenon actually happens in humans who eat a high carbohydrate diet as well.

Animals raised in confined spaces contribute large amounts of manure that must be collected and transported away. This becomes an expensive procedure. It is dumped as close to the feedlot as possible, so there is little cost in removing it. The surrounding areas then become polluted with dangerous bacteria, growth hormones, and antibiotics.

Commercially raised poultry conditions are similar to those of beef. Chickens are raised in crowded pens, often with no access even to fresh air and sunshine. They live packed in a space so small, they can barely move, and eat a diet of grain, hormones and antibiotics. Many chickens are top heavy because they are bred to have lots of 'white meat' and are too weak to stand upright. These poor animals are often trampled and suffocated before they can live out their short and miserable lives.

For all these reasons above, I strictly try to choose healthy grass-fed organic meats… If we're talking about beef or bison, I look for 100% grass-fed (including grass-finished) and organic beef and bison. If it's chicken or turkey, I try to look for free-range, organic birds. Also, wild game is a great option if you have family or friends who are hunters. Wild game will always be some of the healthiest possible meat you can serve yourself and your family.

Some grocery stores are starting to carry better quality meats now, but you can also order meat online on several sites. The one that I personally love and have been using for several years now is http://healthygrassfed.2ya.com. They have amazing quality cuts of meat, as well as some of the best tasting grass-fed burgers I've ever had. They also have a great line of grass-fed sausages (the grass-fed breakfast sausage sliders are amazing!)

Farmed fish vs. wild caught fish

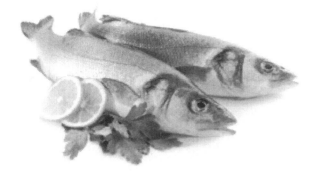

Just as the commercial meat industry in America has now industrialized factory farms producing thousands of pounds of unhealthy meats to meet consumer demand, now there's a similar movement in the global fish farming industry. The fish industry works to satisfy consumers' huge appetites for carnivorous fish, such as salmon, and tuna.

While fish used to be considered a healthy addition to any diet, farmed fish are now barely better than eating a Big Mac and French fries. 'Farmed' fish are not nearly as healthy as wild caught fish in several ways:

• Farmed fish have more fats, but unfortunately it is not the healthy high omega 3 fat that wild fish has.

• Farmed fish are raised in crowded 'feedlot' conditions and, like cattle, need antibiotics to treat the diseases they contract.

• While wild caught salmon have a rosy pink glow indicating they are high in certain antioxidants, farmed salmon are actually an unappetizing grey color, and are fed dye in order to get pink flesh. This dye can actually contain cancer-causing agents.

• Fish farms have a very negative impact on the wild fish population. Toxins, sea lice and other debris from the fish farm ending up killing many of the nearby wild fish.

Nutritional differences of farm-raised vs. wild fish:

Like conventional feedlot cattle, farm-raised fish have more fat. This is not surprising, since farm-raised fish cannot swim through the ocean waters or up clear rocky streams like their wild counterparts. These poor captive fish end up circling lazily in dirty, crowded pens eating an unnatural diet of grain-based fish chow.

Farm-raised fish contain far more omega 6 fatty acids due to their grain-based diet. In fact, farm raised fish have at least twice as much omega 6 fats as wild caught fish do.

While wild ocean fish have low levels of disease and parasites, farm raised fish are rampant with parasites and disease living in densely packed fish farm feedlots. Sea lice, in particular, are one of the worst problems. At the first sign of an outbreak, the fish get pesticides added to their feed.

Farmed salmon and tuna seem to accumulate more cancer-causing PCBs and poisonous dioxins than wild fish. Tests on farmed salmon at grocery stores found 16 times the PCBs compared to wild salmon. Most of these toxins are stored in the fat of the fish, so guess what you are eating when you eat fatty farmed fish?

Fish farms produce an amazing amount of debris, which upsets the balance of the delicate ocean environment. Uneaten feed and fish waste cover the ocean floor beneath these farms, suffocating shellfish and other bottom dwelling sea creatures. An average sized salmon farm produces debris and fish excrement equivalent to the sewage of a city of 10,000 people. Think about that the next time you swim in the ocean! More than half of the fish sold in supermarkets, fish markets, and restaurants are raised on fish farms in the ocean. This exponential growth of the farmed fish industry will continue.

Note that when you're choosing healthier wild caught fish, it is still a good idea to try to limit your intake of fish that are higher on the food chain (tuna, swordfish, shark, striped bass, bluefish) due to the higher levels of mercury in these fish. Fish that are lower on the food chain like sardines, herring, sunfish, trout and salmon have lower levels of mercury and toxins, and are not as much of a concern. Pregnant women should always check with their doctors concerning the types of safe fish to eat.

MEATS/FISH TO AVOID

☐ Packaged, commercially sold grocery store beef (grain-fed) of all cuts

☐ Packaged processed meats like bacon, ham, salami, bologna, hot dogs, sausage, etc (high levels of sodium, nitrates or nitrites, and preservatives).

☐ Frozen prepared meats

☐ Canned meats; processed chipped beef

☐ Regular chicken or turkeys

☐ Canned chicken

☐ Processed chicken or turkey 'lunchmeat'

☐ Frozen snacks with meat or chicken

☐ Any kind of fish that says "farm-raised"

☐ Processed or fried fish such as fish sticks, etc.

☐ Frozen diet dinners

☐ Fast food burgers, fast food fish, fast food chicken, especially "Chicken McNuggets"

By Mike Geary, Certified Personal Trainer, Certified Nutrition Specialist
& Catherine Ebeling – RN, BSN

CHAPTER 9
Soy—Health Food or Frankenfood?

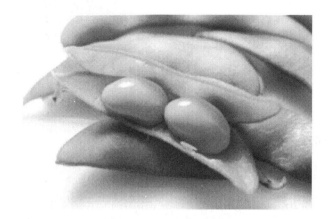

Soy as a health food? Think again! Only a few decades ago, the soybean (un-fermented) was considered unfit to eat—even in Asia where it originated. In western civilizations, it has been considered a "health food."

The soybean, however, was actually not considered edible until the discovery of fermentation techniques. Soy was only eaten as food in a fermented form like tempeh, natto, miso and soy sauce. Unfermented soybeans were never eaten because soybeans contain large quantities of natural toxins which are ac-tually "anti-nutrients". These anti-nutrients block enzymes that are necessary for digestion and absorption of nutrients.

The natural toxins in soy can also produce serious digestive difficulties di-gesting proteins and amino acids. Some of the natural toxins in soybeans are growth inhibitors, and since they block nutrient absorption, children and ba-bies should not eat soy. Soybeans and other legumes contain large amounts of a substance called phytic acid. Phytic acid is found in hulls of many beans or seeds. It blocks essential minerals—calcium, magnesium, copper, iron, and especially zinc from being absorbed.

Soybeans typically contain one of the highest phytate levels of any legume, and even long, slow heating or cooking will not get rid of this substance. Only certain fermenting techniques will remove this nutrient blocker. Phytate con-tent can also be reduced by eating meat with the soy. In many Asian dishes, soy and meat are served together.

If you are a vegetarian, eating tofu and soy products as a substitute for meat and protein may cause you to have nutritional deficiencies. Not only does the risk of B12 deficiency go way up, but mineral deficiencies are common as well. Zinc, calcium, magnesium and iron deficiencies are all very common, but zinc deficiency is often the worst. Sometimes these deficiencies may show up

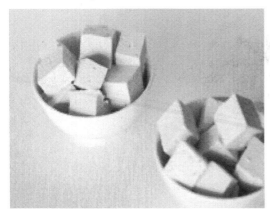 as unnatural cravings for foods like chocolate, and other less-than-healthy foods.

Zinc is necessary for a strong immune system and also plays a role in intelligence and be-havior, because it is needed for proper functioning of the brain and nervous system. Zinc is very im- portant to protein synthesis and collagen formation; it is in-volved in blood-sugar control, and it is needed for a healthy reproductive system.

Soy protein isolate, (SPI) is the often primary protein component in many soy foods, or protein supplements, as well as baby formulas and some brands of soy milk.

What is soy protein isolate? It is not a naturally occurring substance. Soybeans are made into a slurry and combined with an alkaline solution to remove fiber, and then separated using an acid wash, and finally neutralized in an alkaline solution.

The acid washing process happens in aluminum tanks, which leach aluminum into the soy products. Soy curds are then dried at high temperatures to produce a protein powder. This high temperature, high-pressure process then creates TVP or textured vegetable (or soy) protein. But the high temperature process-ing actually denatures the protein, making it virtually useless.

Nitrites (a potent cancer-causing agent) are created in the drying process, and a toxin called lysinoalanine is formed during alkaline processing. Does soy still sound like the healthy super food you thought it was?

Soy protein isolate used to be a waste product of soy processing. Now, it is transformed from unappetizing by-products into something that will be consumed by human beings. Added flavorings, preservatives, sweeteners, emulsi- fiers and synthetic nutrients change soy protein isolate into a seemingly deli- cious manufactured food.

Experiments using soy protein isolate created deficiencies of vitamins E, D, B12, calcium, magnesium, manganese, molybdenum, copper, iron and zinc. The test animals also developed an enlarged pancreas and thyroid gland, and fatty livers.

You don't have to be a vegetarian to be eating soy protein isolate and textured vegetable protein. These products are heavily used in school lunch programs, commercial baked goods, diet foods and fast food products, as well as meat substitutes, protein powders, meal replacement shakes, and energy bars. Many third world countries use soy as a main part of food giveaway programs to starving people.

Soy also contains plant estrogens that disrupt the natural balance of hormones in the body. And if you are a man, do you want to be eating or drinking soy products loaded with substances that mimic female hormones, and lower testosterone? High soy consumption can actually contribute to male breast growth, aka – "man boobs" (gynecomastia). Soy's phytoestrogens can be potentially harmful to women as well, upsetting the delicate natural balance of female hormones.

Soy also seriously interferes with the body's ability to process thyroid hormone, a key protein in metabolism, energy and fat burning ability. Soy is one of the top ten food allergens, and some rate it fifth or sixth highest of allergenic foods. Allergic reactions to soy are increasingly common, ranging from mild to life threatening. And soy is one of the top GMO foods used today, which creates even more health concerns.

Soy is still being marketed to health-conscious consumers, although it is beginning to lose some of its popularity. While the media and soy producers have created an image in the public's mind of soy as a healthy 'natural' superfood, and a supposedly healthy way to escape the so-called evils of saturated fat and cholesterol, in reality, it is far worse. Don't be deceived by clever marketing, soy is not a healthy addition to your diet. Avoid soy.

SOY FOODS TO AVOID

- ☐ Soy Milk
- ☐ Soy baby formula
- ☐ Powdered Soy Protein
- ☐ Protein shakes
- ☐ Tofu
- ☐ Frozen soy "ice cream" products
- ☐ Soy protein energy bars (look at the ingredients as soy protein hides in MOST so-called "energy" bars or protein bars)
- ☐ Textured vegetable protein as an ingredient in meatless products or as a thickener
- ☐ Tofurky
- ☐ Tofu hot dogs
- ☐ MorningStar meatless products
- ☐ Soy snacks, soy chips, soy and rice cake snacks
- ☐ Meatless burgers
- ☐ Meatless fast food meals
- ☐ Edamame (like the kind you get in sushi restaurants)

CHAPTER 10
Sports and Energy Drinks = Sugar + Caffeine

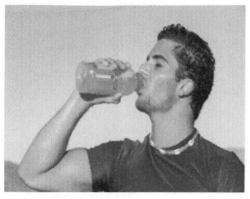

Athletes everywhere reach for sports drinks to quench their thirst and replenish carbohydrates. But do they really work? Do energy and sports drinks help performance or do they just add empty calories?

Creative advertising campaigns and athletic spokespersons give many people the impression that these drinks are healthy and essential during, or after a workout to replace lost electrolytes, carbohydrates and fluids.

Although simple carbohydrates are helpful for athletes engaging in high-intensity exercise, are sports drinks effective, or even appropriate, for the average gym member or weekend warrior?

One study found that citric acid, a common ingredient in sports drinks, ate away the enamel coating on teeth. As a result, the drinks leak into the bone-like material underneath, causing a weakening and softening of the tooth that could result in severe tooth damage, cavities, and even tooth loss if left untreated.

Sports drinks can be up to 30 times more erosive to your teeth than water. As a recent study pointed out, brushing your teeth will not help remove the citric acid. It softens tooth enamel so much that brushing causes further damage. So, sports drinks can lead to serious dental problems!

According to researchers at the University of New Mexico, "unless a person is going to exercise for at least 90 minutes, consuming the sugar in the drinks is pointless." While sports drinks containing sugar or fructose may help the body absorb water, there's no evidence that your body will retain water more effectively than if you just drank water alone so they are not more effective at battling dehydration.

The leading brands of sports drinks on the market typically contain as much sugar as sodas and more sodium. They also often contain high-fructose corn syrup (HFCS), artificial flavors, and food coloring, none of which belong in your body, and none of which are healthy. In another study on fructose (as in high fructose corn syrup), vs. regular sugar, it was found that the fructose is metabolized by the liver and converted immediately into fats or triglycerides, stored as fat, and not even burned for energy.

If you are exercising to lose weight and get into shape, you should know that sports drinks and energy drinks will cause weight gain, similar to drinking soda. It's a sad irony that many people work hard to lose weight, only to gain it back from drinking sports drinks.

Although these drinks are often referred to as "energy" drinks, in the long run the sugar they contain does just the opposite. Blood sugar plummets following the quick explosion of energy, as your system floods with insulin. The insulin takes your body out of the fat burning zone and right into the fat storing zone. Soon, the quick energy you got from the sugar fizzles out, as 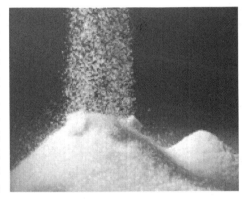 your blood sugar drops. And lo and behold, hunger cravings start as soon as the blood sugar drops.

Fructose converts to fat more quickly and efficiently than any other sugar, and raises your triglycerides (circulating fats in the blood stream) significantly. To convert fructose into glucose it must rob ATP energy stores from the liver. ATP is the fuel which supplies the energy to muscles, especially while exercising. If you are robbing your muscles' energy stores, then your sports drink is actually *decreasing* your athletic performance! So now you are tired and weaker from drinking sports drinks...

If your sports drink is low calorie and sugar-free, then it most likely contains an artificial sweetener, which is even worse for you than high-fructose corn syrup or sugar. And don't think that because a sport drink claims to be low-or no-calorie that it won't contribute to weight gain. As mentioned before, arti-

Maximize Your Flat Belly Journey: Get Powerful Fat Loss Secrets From Key Food And Fitness Experts.
http://velocityhousepresents.com/FlatBellyKitchen

ficial sweeteners are as big a culprit in weight gain as sugar and corn syrup.

Sports drinks also contain large quantities of salt, which is there to replace electrolytes. But, unless you're sweating profusely and for a prolonged period, that extra salt is simply unnecessary, and possibly harmful. Too many concentrated electrolytes can actually throw off your body's own delicate electrolyte balance. The excess salt will actually make you thirstier and make you want to drink more, while causing you to retain water and feel heavier and look bloated. While you may think you are doing your body good, drinking sports drinks is no better than drinking soda after your workout.

Energy drinks were popularized in the U.S. with the introduction of Red Bull®, a carbonated beverage from Austria that contains 80 mg of caffeine per serving—about the same amount as is found in a cup of coffee. For comparison, classic Coca Cola® contains 23 mg caffeine and Mountain Dew® contains 37 mg caffeine. Other brands of energy drinks may contain twice as much or more caffeine as Red Bull.

The calories in these drinks do provide some energy, but mostly their content of caffeine, guarana, and taurine increase feelings of alertness, but may also produce troublesome side effects such as anxiety, irritability, heart palpitations, difficulty sleeping, and indigestion. These occurrences are more likely to happen with energy drinks than with coffee, which we generally sip, versus chugging chilled energy drinks. Energy drinks can also lead to dehydration because the caffeine stimulates urination and thus increases water and electrolyte loss. Dehydration during athletic activities not only drastically reduces performance, but also can cause painful muscle cramping.

This is the bottom line: Any workout less than an hour or so will not result in a large enough fluid loss to justify using these high-sodium, high-sugar drinks. It's only when you've been exercising for longer periods, such as 90 minutes or more, or at an extreme intensity, such as on a very hot day, or going 100%, that you may need something more than water to replenish your body. Less than 1 percent of those who use sports drinks actually benefit from them. Keep burning fat and drink water!

If you do workout in the heat for several hours, consider using a healthier natural drink such as pure 100% coconut water instead of processed sugar-laden sports drinks. Coconut water is delicious and can have as much as 1000 mg of potassium per 20 oz drink.

SPORTS/ENERGY DRINKS TO AVOID

- Gatorade, all kinds
- Powerade
- Red Bull
- Monster
- Rock Star
- 5 Hour Energy
- AMP
- Bulldog
- Bawls
- Fuse
- Sobe Adrenalin Rush
- TAB Energy
- Vault
- Snapple
- And many more

Maximize Your Flat Belly Journey: Get Powerful Fat Loss Secrets From Key Food And Fitness Experts.
http://velocityhousepresents.com/FlatBellyKitchen

By Mike Geary, Certified Personal Trainer, Certified Nutrition Specialist
& Catherine Ebeling – RN, BSN

CHAPTER 11
Energy Bars, Protein Bars or, Glorified Candy Bars?

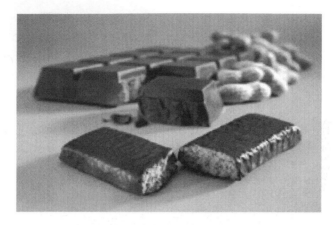

They claim to be healthy, contain protein and fiber, advertised to contain vitamins and minerals, but look and taste like candy bars. And, they are convenient and taste good. Somehow we have been duped into thinking this is a healthy snack food or worse yet, a meal replacement. And if you browse the energy bar shelves at your grocery store, you will see that more and more varieties appear every day. We'll show you at the end of this section that there are a few rare healthy energy bars, but most are just candy bars in disguise.

The original energy bars, like the Power Bar and the Source Bar, were based on so-called 'natural' sweeteners—high fructose corn syrup and juice concentrates—along with dried fruits and nuts, a combination that resulted in higher percentages of carbohydrates than the typical chocolate candy bar (which is rich in cocoa butter, a healthy natural fat.)

When cheap soy and whey proteins became available, the energy bar industry exploded. Protein was added to make a 'high-protein' bar. Balance Bars ("The Complete Nutritional Food Bar") and ZonePerfect Bars ("All Natural Nutrition Bars"), and Atkins Bars were among the first to hit the shelves as energy/ protein bars.

But there is nothing natural about the protein used in today's energy bars. Most bars contain highly processed soy protein (see the previous chapter on soy products). Isolated soy protein comes with an initial burden of

nutrient-blocking agents such as phytic acid, enzyme inhibitors and iso-flavones. Much of the soy in energy bars is genetically modified, as well.

More toxins are formed during high-temperature, high-pressure chemical processing, including nitrates, lysinalanine and MSG. Soy protein is processed at very high temperatures to reduce the levels of phytic acid and enzyme inhibitors. This process degrades most of protein in soy, making it virtually useless as usable protein in the body.

The other frequently used protein is whey protein, which must be processed at low temperatures or the protein is damaged from a nutritional standpoint. When cheese, butter, and cream were produced on farms in the past, the leftover whey and skim milk used to be given to the pigs and chickens. Now the dairy industry has an overabundance of whey, solved by drying it at high temperatures and putting the powders into protein drinks, bodybuilding powders and high-protein bars. The delicate protein molecules in the processed whey are damaged and denatured by heat processing, and the quality of the protein is lacking.

Remember that if you use whey protein for your smoothies or other recipes, I recommend a cold-processed, grass-fed whey protein from cows that are raised in a healthy manner instead of on commercial factory farms. This is my favorite grass-fed whey I've been using for a couple years now: http://BestGrassFedWhey.com

Other major ingredients in energy bars include high fructose corn syrup, an ingredient that we've established is worse than sugar. And in humans, it causes our insulin levels to spike as the fructose hits our livers, and is immediately processed into fat particles and stored as body fat. Energy bars also include fiber from oats, apples, soy, and citrus. Sometimes maltodextrin is given as the fiber source. "Natural flavors" and piles of synthetic vitamins are thrown in so the bars can be called "complete."

On the good side, the fat source in most energy bars is often palm, palm kernel, or coconut oil, and so they are generally healthier for you than hydrogenated oils and trans fats (or other heavily refined omega 6 oils).

So, with the exception of the fats, most of the ingredients used in energy bars are industrial food waste products—soy protein isolate and whey protein are the waste by-products of the soy and dairy industries. Apple and lemon fiber, often used to create a crunchy effect, are also waste, made from the pulp left over from squeezing the fruits for their juice. Soy lecithin, another common ingredient, is also a waste product of the soy industry. So you see, the ingredients are mostly food waste by-products and are anything but natural!

While many of the modern energy bars emphasize athletic performance, others claim to promote optimal mental performance. No energy bar/protein bar that you can eat will optimize your athletic performance, or mental performance over eating real food. You just cannot do it. The energy bar phenomenon capitalizes on a real human need—that of a convenient, nutrient-dense, concentrated food that travels well, and doesn't spoil, satisfies, and tastes good.

My best advice: ignore the hype and advertising of the slick, packaged energy bars. These bars are not healthy food, they are candy bars—or worse—disguised as something the big food companies will tell you can substitute for meals, pump up your energy, or help you improve your athletic performance.

There are better alternatives. Only REAL food will build up your body, fuel your energy and enhance your health. Stick to unprocessed, unpackaged food that has few ingredients. Your body will thank you for it.

Some good alternatives to energy bars for quick healthy snacks on the go could be as simple as a bag of mixed raw nuts (almonds, pecans, walnuts, etc) with a little bit of dried fruit (just beware of eating large amounts of dried fruit due to the high sugar content). Check out the recipe for Natural Nutty Snacks at the end of the chapter on nuts. They are a great substitute for energy bars!

If you want to try one of the healthiest bars I've tried recently, check out Dale's raw protein bars. Each Raw Protein Bar has between 240-280 calories, 22g protein, 12-28g carbs (7-8g fiber), and 12-16g of healthy fat.

My favorites are:

-Blueberry Macadamia
-Strawberry Banana
-Raspberry Hazelnut

-Chocolate Chia Maca
-and Low-Carb Cafe Mocha

Really good stuff! Warning though... beware of the "Goji and greens" flavor... both my girlfriend and I were NOT fans of this flavor. But the other five that I listed above we really loved! You can grab some of these tasty Raw Protein bars here.

THE WORST ENERGY BARS

- ☐ Luna Bars

- ☐ Kashi GoLean

- ☐ Powerbars

- ☐ Quaker Chewy Granola bars

- ☐ Kudos

- ☐ MetRx

- ☐ Balance bars

- ☐ Clif Bars, Builder, Crunch, Mojo

- ☐ Genisoy

- ☐ Snickers Marathon

- ☐ Soy Sensations

- ☐ Anything with high fructose corn syrup, lots of sugar, refined flours, isolated soy protein or any other unidentifiable ingredients

CHAPTER 12
Diet Food, Frozen Weight Loss Meals, and Low Fat Foods

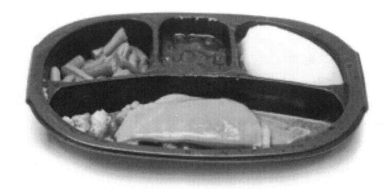

There are many chemicals and flavor enhancers in processed foods and those so-called 'diet' foods that are packaged as weight loss dinners, desserts, snacks, etc., and many of those are addictive. MSG is one good example. People who eat monosodium glutamate, or MSG, as a flavor enhancer in their food are more likely to be overweight or obese even with the same amount of physical activity and caloric intake, as others not eating MSG, according to a University of North Carolina at Chapel Hill School of Public Health.

The bottom line is that you should avoid MSG as much as possible since it stimulates cravings and leads to weight gain. The best way to avoid MSG is simply to avoid all processed foods. For some people, that may sound difficult, but it really becomes simple if the only foods that you buy at the grocery store are 1-ingredient foods – that means fresh whole unprocessed foods.

Most low-calorie foods cut calories by removing refined cane sugar and replacing it with artificial sweeteners like Aspartame, Sweet'n'Low, Splenda, and a dozen other sugar-like compounds. These artificial sweeteners contain less (in some cases, zero) calories, but they are incredibly dangerous in other ways, as we've already discussed, and contribute to weight gain, not weight loss.

Artificial sweeteners have been linked to cancer, migraines, depression, birth defects, infertility, seizures, thyroid problems, and weight gain. In addition, low-calorie diet foods are usually loaded with processed ingredients that the body doesn't know what to do with, so it stores these ingredients as wastes in fat stores within the body.

Among the most common processed ingredients are refined/enriched flours, starches and fillers (corn starch), colors, preservatives (which go by hundreds of different names), and chemical flavorings, which may legally be called "natural flavors" even if they include MSG. (As a side note: most varieties of processed or "textured" soy protein, TSP or TVP, use MSG for flavor and call it "natural flavors").

The array of starches, fillers, artificial flavors, high fructose corn syrup, preservatives, chemicals and unhealthy fats not only make it hard for the body to find any useable nutrition, but they wreak havoc on your system. All these unnatural ingredients contain chemicals that can mess with brain and nervous function, causing mental and emotional issues, irritability, sleepiness, weakness and fatigue.

All this processed food contributes to inflammation in the body, causing fluid buildup, puffiness, and weight gain. And inflammation, as you know, is the beginning point for many serious diseases including cancer, many autoimmune diseases, and heart disease, to name just a few.

Many nutrition experts believe that the more refined a food is, the less satisfying it is to the body. Because the body is unable to extract the nutrients it needs from denatured, highly processed junk foods; it craves more nourishment. Cravings are usually a signal your body is not getting the nutrients it needs. However, sugars and starches stimulate appetite and increase cravings for sugar—as do most artificial sweeteners.

Even the best food companies, whose apparent goal is to promote health and wellness, are still in business to make a profit. Corporations selling diet foods and low-cal foods are hardly motivated to make a product that really helps people consume less and lose weight. If they did, their repeat buyers—people who are overweight—would disappear, taking their money with them.

Weight loss products are highly suspect for their harmful and addictive artificial ingredients, and for the elusive promise of "quick, easy" weight loss they promise but almost never fulfill. Don't be fooled by the pretty pictures, the convincing advertising and the promises to help you lose weight. None of it is true. This stuff is not 'real' food, and it will do nothing but make you gain weight, feel terrible, and cause a myriad of health problems.

The only certain way to lose weight permanently is to focus on healthy REAL food, such as organic fruits and vegetables, raw nuts and seeds, grass-fed meats, free range poultry and raw dairy products, an active lifestyle, reducing stress, and creating balance and harmony in our lives.

PROCESSED, PACKAGED, REFINED "DIET FOOD" (FAT FUEL, AS I CALL IT) TO AVOID

- ☐ Weight Watchers dinners, Lean Cuisine, SmartOnes, Healthy Choice, Kid Cuisine

- ☐ Cool Whip Lite, Cool Whip Free, Cool Whip sugar-free, or any other imtation whipped cream

- ☐ Sugar free popsicles, sugar-free ice cream treats

- ☐ Sugar free or fat free desserts, cookies, cakes, etc.

- ☐ Slim Fast (or other brands) diet shakes/meal replacements, snack bars, powder mix

- ☐ Instant Breakfast

- ☐ Fiber One, Pop Tarts, cookies, muffins, etc.

- ☐ Special K Bars

- ☐ Rice cakes

- ☐ Anything packaged, processed or with the words, "Low fat," "Sugar free," "Fat free," "Diet," etc.

PART TWO

Creating Your Flat Belly Kitchen

Maximize Your Flat Belly Journey: Get Powerful Fat Loss Secrets From Key Food And Fitness Experts.
http://velocityhousepresents.com/FlatBellyKitchen

CHAPTER 13
In Search of High Quality Protein

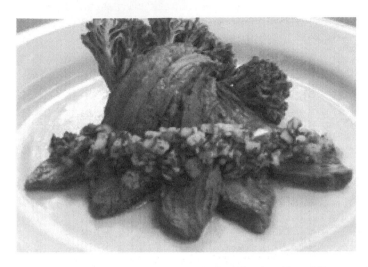

Protein often is lumped into a generic group all by itself. While protein is extremely important as a macronutrient, the source of the protein is extremely crucial. All protein is not equal. With the current health issues of obesity, diabetes, and the aging population, getting high quality, useable protein has never been more important.

Many body builders will have you believe that the more protein you get the better. In terms of weight loss, lean body composition and weight maintenance, there is much more to the story than that.

Eating the right balance of protein from the right sources can help your body maintain stable blood sugar levels and keep you from being hungry as often. Protein helps promote a feeling of fullness, and because it doesn't stimulate your insulin release, it can help to prevent cravings for starchy, sugary snacks. We all know that protein is a building block and it is very true. Protein is put to use by the body in building muscles, it is stored for energy, and the amino acids are used throughout the body for various essential functions, such as supplying energy and supporting healthy brain function.

Health and fitness professionals often debate over how much protein is necessary for good health, to build or maintain muscle, or just to lose weight. I've heard every argument on both sides of this equation, including many experts who insist that we only need small amounts of protein daily… but I always come back to the anecdotal evidence I've observed over the years and I can't ignore this evidence.

I've known dozens of fitness models, bodybuilders, and athletes with incredible physiques over the years, and one common thread I've always noticed with the people that have the absolute best bodies is that they include a high amount of protein in their diet – higher than typical recommended amounts. In fact, I've even questioned several fitness models on what they think is one of the most important parts of their dietary regimen, and they consistently mention protein intake first. Again, this is only anecdotal evidence, and every person has unique needs.

So, if you begin by increasing your daily protein intake beyond the Recommended Dietary Allowance (RDA) of 0.8 g/kg/day, you will find this may enhance muscle development and help to reduce progressive loss of muscle mass with age (sarcopenia).

Most fitness experts go by the general rule of 1 gram of protein per pound of bodyweight per day (that would be over 2 grams of protein per KG of bodyweight per day). But this estimate has flaws too, as an obese individual would certainly never need extreme amounts of protein to equal 1 gram per lb of bodyweight, and the excess protein would actually be stored as fat.

The bottom line is that there is no magical ratio of protein that is "perfect" for you. If you're getting 20-30 grams of protein per meal from quality sources, and eating 5-6 small meals/day, that is going to provide all of the protein that most normal sized people would need.

Besides creating a lean strong body, diets containing increased protein portions and reduced carbohydrates have positive effects in treating or preventing type 2 diabetes and reducing risk factors for coronary heart disease. High-quality protein plays an increasingly important role in weight management, muscle development and maintenance, as well as general disease prevention.

Good quality protein is key to your body's ability to use it. Real protein is far better than manufactured protein powders. High quality grass-fed beef or bison, free range chicken and organic eggs, and wild caught fish are the best protein sources you can eat. These protein sources contain the right ratios of omega 3 fats to omega 6 fats, and contain highly bio-available protein that is easier to digest and assimilate than commercially raised livestock and poultry.

In addition, omega 3 fats in grass-fed meats and wild caught fish are essential to optimal health and improve your cells' response to insulin, neurotransmitters and other messengers. They're also very important for the repair process of damaged cells. When your body is deprived of important essential fats like omega 3's, your metabolic rate slows down, so you can't burn calories as efficiently. In fact, weight gain and inflammation are two key symptoms of omega 3 deficiency.

The best types of meat protein are free of hormones, antibiotics and toxins; meaning they are considered 'clean' proteins, with no toxic residue to be stored in your tissues. Toxins stored in your body's fat will make it harder to lose that fat, once you start trying to change your diet. So stick to 'clean' proteins with the highest quality protein you can get. Sure it does cost a little more, but your body is utilizing more of the protein and getting loads more nutrition from it! So actually you are getting more for your money this way.

Grass-fed Beef or Bison

Ok, so you may have been told that beef is evil, bad for your health, loaded with saturated fats, and fattening. Forget that. This is a whole different animal than you are used to. Red meat may have a bad reputation, but there is a healthier type of red meat than the commercially raised red meat you get from the grocery store. 100% grass-fed meat is a far better choice, and is one of the best, most usable forms of high quality fat burning, muscle building protein you can eat.

The large amounts of nutrients that grass-fed cattle and bison consume in their daily diet are passed on to you. Grass-fed meats are very different than commercially raised meats from the grocery store. Grass-fed meats are a totally different animal, so to speak.

70

Grass-fed beef and bison contain far more healthy usable protein in the form of branch chain amino acids, iron, beta-carotene (vitamin A), vitamin E, conjugated linoleic acid (CLA), and omega 3 fatty acids than grain-fed (conventional) meat. Grass-fed meat aids fat burning and muscle building processes, as well as containing many micronutrients, and antioxidants.

Three ounces of ground beef from regular grain-fed cattle contains about 40 micrograms of beta-carotene. Grass-fed meat has more than DOUBLE the beta-carotene at 87 micrograms for 3 ounces of ground beef. Beta-carotene is what the body uses to make vitamin A.

Vitamin A is a vital fat-soluble vitamin that is important for vision, bone growth, reproduction, cell division, immune function, and energy production. Grass-fed meats are much higher in Vitamin E. Vitamin E is another fat-soluble vitamin with powerful antioxidant activity. Grass-fed cattle contain about 3 times as much vitamin E per serving as conventional beef!

But here is the most important thing to keep in mind about grass-fed meat—the fat content and the fat ratios. Grass-fed meat has about 30% less fat per serving and the fat it does contain is far healthier for you—in fact, it is essential to your health.

Some fats are actually very important to help with weight loss and maintaining good health. We need a certain group of fats called essential fatty acids (EFAs), which must be obtained from the food that we eat. Grass-fed meat has significantly higher levels of omega 3 essential fatty acids, and Conjugated Linoleic Acid (CLA)—both known for their ability to help in fat-burning, muscle building, fighting inflammation, and good general health (including for cancer risk reduction, diabetes protection, healthy pregnancies, heart disease risk reduction, etc).

Meat from cattle raised on 100% grass have somewhere around 60% more omega 3 fatty acids, and a much better omega 6 to omega 3 ratio. And as we discussed in earlier chapters, we need far more omega 3 fats and far less omega 6 fats than most people currently eat on a modern western diet.

The latest research has linked higher blood levels of the omega 3 fatty acids, EPA and DHA, to lower rates of obesity. A recent study found people with higher omega 3 blood levels had lower Body Mass Indexes, narrower waists, and smaller hip circumferences. The study suggests that omega 3 supplementation may play an important role in preventing weight gain and improving weight loss when supplemented with a structured weight-loss program.

Omega 3s may increase the burning of body fat by the process known as thermogenesis, in which oxidation of body fat burns it off in the form of body heat. Omega 3 fatty acids activate the enzymes responsible for burning fat, and combined with exercise, they increase the metabolic rate, which has an effect of burning more fat and losing weight.

One human study found that omega 3s boosted the feeling of fullness after a meal, among overweight and obese people participating in a weight loss program.

Another key reason why omega 3 fatty acids have such a powerful effect on fat metabolism is that insulin levels are lowered when subjects are eating more omega 3s. By lowering insulin levels, you keep the body burning fat for energy instead of storing fat.

In addition, omega 3 oils have many other positive benefits, including improving acne, and smoothing wrinkles, lowering inflammation levels in the body, and reducing the effects of autoimmune diseases. Omega 3s also reduce the risk of heart disease and stroke while helping to reduce symptoms of hypertension, depression, attention deficit hyperactivity disorder (ADHD), joint pain and arthritis, as well as certain skin ailments.

Some research has even shown that omega 3s boost the immune system and help protect the brain and nervous system, as well as protecting from a variety of illnesses including Alzheimer's disease, multiple sclerosis, and cancer. And for women who are pregnant or trying to get pregnant, omega 3s are extremely helpful for a developing a fetus' brain and nerves. In fact, omega 3 fatty acids may actually improve your child's learning ability and intelligence.

The meat and milk from grass-fed cattle and bison are the richest known source of another type of essential fat called "conjugated linoleic acid" or CLA. When cattle are raised on grass or hay, and not grains, their milk and meat contain as much as five times more CLA than products from animals fed conventional diets.

What exactly is CLA? CLA is a type of fat that has been proven in scientific studies in recent years to help metabolize and burn fat, and build muscle (which means eating more of this type of healthy fat will actually help you get lean and ripped!). These benefits are on top of the fact that grass-fed meats are some of the highest quality proteins that you can possibly eat—easily digestible and easily utilized by your body.

In addition, CLA may be one of the best defenses against cancer. Yes, a fat that helps fight cancer! In studies, scientists have shown that CLA can lower an individual's risk for cancer and arteriosclerosis, as well as reducing body fat and delaying the onset of diabetes. So while it is making your body stronger and leaner, it is also protecting you from deadly diseases.

CLA has become so valued for its health benefits that many health food stores sell CLA supplements, but naturally occurring CLA is utilized much more effectively by the body than these synthetic supplements, which are prone to oxidation during shelf life.

Grass-fed lamb, and goat has similar high quality protein and healthy fats as grass-fed beef and bison. Ostrich meat and venison are other healthy meats full of great nutrition too. So get adventurous and try something exotic!

One other great added benefit of grass-fed meat from healthy animals is that dangerous E.coli does not thrive in a healthy grass-fed animal! When cattle are fed a diet of grains, it increases the amount of acid in their stomachs while they are trying to digest that unnatural diet. Increased acid and the drastic change in pH in cattle is the breeding ground for the dangerous E.coli bacteria that sickens and kills people. When grass-fed cattle eat their natural diet, E.coli bacteria cannot grow in this environment. Why mess with Mother Nature? Grass-fed meat is not only better for you, but safer too!

Be sure to always choose 100% grass-fed meat. Meat that is 'finished' on grain does not have the same health benefits of entirely grass-fed meats.

Grass-fed meats are harder to find in most grocery stores, but one place online that we found a wide variety of delicious grass-fed meats (steaks, burgers, specialty meats, etc) delivered right to your door is at this website: http://healthy-grassfed.2ya.com/

One of the best high protein snacks is pure, all-natural grass-fed beef jerky. This is an easy and relatively inexpensive way to get good quality protein when you just need a little something. And beef jerky is a great concentrated source of lean protein, plus all the benefits of grass-fed meat.

Wild Caught Fish

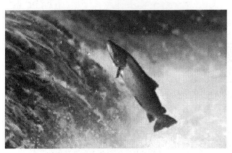 The BIG factor in both wild caught fish and grass-fed meats is the type of fat and the fat ratios. Like grass-fed meat, the fats in wild caught fish are especially healthy. Both have significantly higher levels of the essential fatty acid omega 3, which has powerfully positive effects in your body.

Like beef, the fat composition in farmed fish changes drastically when fed a grain-based diet and kept in pens, so stick to wild caught fish. Wild caught fish eating their natural diet have the ideal fat composition—high in fat-burning healthy omega 3s and lower in inflammatory omega 6s. We know the benefits of omega 3s have on our bodies, so eating wild caught fish is the best choice.

Unless you've been living under a rock somewhere for the last several years, you've probably heard about the health benefits of eating fatty fish or taking fish oil supplements. Well, add fat loss to the other benefits like heart, blood (cholesterol/triglycerides), brain, skin and joint health (and the rest of the list which is too long to print here). The active ingredients that seem to make fatty fish so beneficial are the omega 3 fatty acids, EPA and DHA. Omega 3 fatty acids are very beneficial in helping the body lose fat.

What about mercury in fish? Mercury in fish occurs in some of the higher food chain predatory fish such as tuna and swordfish. Even though they are higher in the good fats, they also store a considerable amount of mercury and other toxins in their fat. Mercury is very detrimental to the brain and overall health, and is a neurotoxin that is difficult for the body to eliminate.

What is the best type of wild caught fish to eat? Everybody knows about salmon (wild salmon, of course, not farm raised) being a great source of omega 3 fatty acids, and clean protein, so that choice comes as no big surprise. What are our other good choices? Wild caught halibut and wild cod are great fish full of omega 3s as well.

Another great high omega 3 fish alternative that doesn't have the issues with mercury that tuna, swordfish, and other larger fish do, is sardines—of all things! Before you think, "Eww, I don't like sardines!" it might be time to want to give them another look—or taste.

Sardines are a great choice for a quick healthy meal—tons of muscle-building appetite satisfying protein; super high in healthy omega 3 healthy fats, and much lower in mercury and other pollutants than most fish.

One of the benefits of sardines is their generous amount of omega 3 fats, such as EPA and DHA—which are far superior than eating plant-based omega 3 fats for example, from flaxseeds or walnuts, where your body still needs to try to convert the shorter chain omega 3s to longer chain omega 3s. This is an in efficient conversion, so one of the best ways to provide your body with the important EPA and DHA is through fatty wild caught fish, fish oil, or krill oil.

The type of dietary fat (monounsaturated, saturated, or polyunsaturated) we consume alters the production of a group of biological compounds known as eicosanoids in our bodies. These eicosanoids have a significant biological influence on blood pressure, blood clotting, inflammation, immune function, and heart function.

One of the important things to remember about inflammatory processes is weight gain. Also, the lack of ability to lose weight is a major sign of inflammation. So reducing inflammation is always a key factor in fat loss! Omega 3 oils also have additional protective effects against heart disease by:

- Decreasing blood lipids (cholesterol, LDL, and triglycerides)

- Decreasing blood clotting factors in the vascular system

- Increasing relaxation in larger arteries and other blood vessels

- Decreasing inflammatory processes in blood vessels, which leads to plaque buildup on arterial walls

Other studies have provided good news about the benefits of omega 3 oils for individuals with arthritis, psoriasis, ulcerative colitis, lupus, asthma, and certain cancers—all diseases related to inflammation.

Most people with inflammatory health problems at some point have to resort to steroid-based drugs if they are not stringent about their diet. The effect of steroids on the body is to cause immediate (and very difficult to lose) weight gain, facial puffiness and appetite increase. Avoiding the use of these heavy duty drugs will go a long way towards your weight loss goals, and getting the lean, ripped body you are striving for!

Wild caught fatty fish is also an excellent source of natural vitamin E, a powerful antioxidant. Antioxidants, which also include vitamin C and beta-carotene, deactivate harmful free radicals. Vitamin E also lowers the risk of heart disease by preventing the oxidation of low-density lipoproteins (LDLs or the 'bad' cholesterol), and helping prevent buildup of plaque in coronary arteries.

As far as taste is concerned, there is no comparison. Wild fish has a much better taste and texture, and the meat does not get a bad, "fishy" smell or taste that farmed fish is known to have. Just keep in mind that wild caught fish have a firmer texture and may be slightly drier, so be careful not to overcook it.

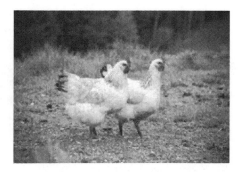

Free Range Chicken

Free range chicken is becoming much more popular and easier to find. Not only is the taste better, but the health benefits are much better than factory farm-raised chicken. Quite simply, free range chickens make for healthier, better tasting meat. When animals are cared for properly, and given a supportive, all-natural environment in which to live, the food they yield is better for you and full of the nutrients you need.

There's more, however, to the notion of free range and all natural chicken than simply making the animal happy and healthy. It's a health issue for you, the consumer!

The case for free range chickens is becoming a stronger one for so many reasons, and we, the meat buying public, are becoming more and more health conscious and aware of its importance. Most of us know about the antibiotics and hormones the animals are given.

The conditions under which meat-producing animals are raised play a large role as well. Commercially raised chickens live in very close quarters where they can hardly move or turn around. They are fed hormone-enhanced grain and antibiotics and fattened up as quickly as possible.

On the other hand, free range chickens roam outside in their natural environment with sun and fresh air, and eat what they need at will. They eat a natural diet, including the things that keep the good fat ratios (omega 3 to omega 6) in the healthy range—similar to wild caught fish and grass-fed meats.

Most free range, organically raised chickens do not need antibiotics or artificial growth hormones. They eat healthy, vegetarian feed, and roam around and eat greens, bugs, worms, and grubs, which is an important part of their natural diet. This increases the fat-burning omega 3s in their meat and their eggs.

Chicken meat has a naturally lower fat percentage than most red meats, but again it is best to purchase the free range, organically-raised kind. Otherwise, avoid eating the skin, which stores the largest amount of bad fats, hormones, antibiotics and other toxins.

Keep some cooked up chicken breasts on hand to throw into wraps with some lettuce and avocado for a delicious, quick and filling eat-on-the-run meal.

Whole Organic Free range Eggs

By Mike Geary, Certified Personal Trainer, Certified Nutrition Specialist
& Catherine Ebeling – RN, BSN

Whole Eggs, including the yolk (not just egg whites) are an incredibly good source of usable protein. Most people know that eggs are one of the highest quality sources of protein. However, most people don't know that the egg yolks are the healthiest part of the egg. That's where we find almost all of the vitamins, minerals, and antioxidants (such as lutein).

Egg yolks contain more than 90% of the calcium, iron, phosphorus, zinc, thiamin, B6, folate, and B12, and panthothenic acid of the egg. In addition, the yolks contain ALL of the fat-soluble vitamins A, D, E, and K in the egg, as well as ALL of the essential fatty acids. Also, the protein of whole eggs is more bio-available than egg whites alone due to a more balanced amino acid profile that the yolks help to build.

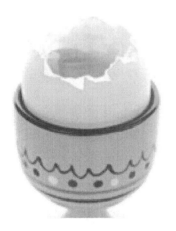

Just make sure to choose free range organic eggs instead of normal grocery store eggs. Similar to the grass-fed beef scenario, the nutrient content of the eggs and the balance between healthy omega 3 fatty acids and inflammatory omega 6 fatty acids (in excess) depends on the diet of the chickens.

Chickens that roam free outside and eat a more natural diet will give you healthier, more nutrient-rich eggs with a healthier

fat balance compared with your typical grocery store eggs (that came from chickens fed nothing but soy and corn and kept in crowded, dirty "egg factories" all day long).

Eggs from pastured free range hens can contain up 10x more omega 3 fatty acids compared to eggs from factory farmed hens. FYI – some companies may claim on the egg cartons that their hens are "free range," but some companies only let their hens outside for 5 or 10 minutes per day, and can fit into this category. This is a far cry from truly free range pastured hens that spend most of their time outside in a given day.

Your best bet is to get eggs from a local farmer or co-op where you know for certain how the chickens have been raised. If you can't find a co-op, farmer's market, or farm near you, and you are forced to get your eggs from the grocery store, choose organic and free-range. In most instances, these will be higher quality eggs with more nutrition than typical factory farmed eggs.

Eggs are such a versatile food; you can scramble them and throw in veggies to make an omelet, or boil to take with you for a great high protein snack. I like to keep a few boiled eggs on hand to throw into a salad or sandwiches, or grated on top of soups or veggies.

Throw an egg into your smoothie for added protein, or add egg to your stir-fry.

CHAPTER 14
The Real Story on Raw Dairy

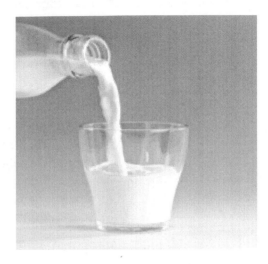

Milk and dairy products sometimes get a bad rap. For regular commercially produced pasteurized, homogenized dairy products, it's probably true. Hormones, antibiotics, and white blood cells (pus, left over from udder infections) all end up in the milk you buy from the grocery store. It is heated to the point that all the vital enzymes and most of the nutrients are killed. The milk proteins become distorted from the heat, and it becomes hard to digest and causes allergic reactions.

It isn't much other than a white, fattening liquid at that point. Even if you purchase organic milk, while you do avoid the hormones and antibiotics to some extent, you are still missing out on a lot of important nutrients, since it is still pasteurized.

On the other hand, raw milk—especially milk from grass-fed cows is a whole other story! As we mentioned in Part 1, raw milk (unpasteurized, unhomogenized) from healthy grass-fed cows is the only source of milk that can be considered healthy. Did you know that clean, raw milk from grass-fed cows was actually used as a medicine in the early part of the last century? It's true.

Clean, raw milk was used as medicine to treat serious chronic diseases. From the days of Hippocrates to until just after World War II, this miracle food has been used to nourish and heal. Did you know that you could actually live exclusively on clean, raw milk, butter and cheese, if you had to? Raw dairy contains a wealth of healthy bodybuilding and fat burning, flat belly substances including: amino acids, enzymes, vitamins, minerals, and healthy fats, including omega 3 fats and CLA (conjugated linoleic acid).

Amino acids are the building blocks for protein. We use somewhere around 20-22 of them for protein construction, which builds muscle. Raw dairy contains 20 of these necessary amino acids. About 80% of the proteins in milk are from caseins, and the other 20% of the proteins are classified as whey proteins, which are very heat sensitive. Along with these protein sources, raw milk contains some very important enzymes, (which help the body digest and assimilate the nutrient in milk) immunoglobulins (key immune factors), vitamin binding proteins and growth factors.

About two-thirds of the fat in milk is saturated. While many of us think that saturated fat is bad for us, this is just not true. Saturated fats are actually necessary for proper body function and are a part of healthy cell membranes, and our hormones. In addition, they supply the brain with the fats it needs to function properly and serve as a vehicle for fat-soluble vitamins.

Saturated fats also cause the stomach lining to secrete a hormone which stimulates secretion of digestive enzymes, and signal the brain that we've eaten enough. This is why non-fat dairy and other fat-free foods can cause over-eating; there is no fat to signal the brain to stop.

Grass-fed dairy has one of the highest amounts of Conjugated Linoleic Acid (CLA) of any foods. Among CLA's many benefits include raising your metabolic rate, which means you burn more fat, it helps eliminate belly fat, boosts muscle growth, reduces insulin resistance, strengthens the immune system, and lowers food allergy reactions. And remember this about grass-fed raw dairy over conventional dairy: it contains about 5 times more CLA than the poor quality milk you buy at your local grocery store! Raw milk also has some key superstar ingredients that not only benefit your health, but also keep the milk safe for you to drink:

Lactoferrin is an iron-binding protein found in raw milk. It's an effective antioxidant, anti-fungal, antibacterial, antiviral, anti-inflammatory, anti-cancer agent and immune-boosting powerhouse. Lactoferrin is so powerful, it can kill the dangerous form of E.coli bacteria, which is capable of making humans very ill. Heating, as in pasteurization, destroys its ability to kill harmful bacteria that may enter the milk. Two other raw milk ingredients also kill off unwanted bacteria and pathogens. These are lysozyme, and lactoperoxidase. These immune-enhancing substances, along with immunoglobulin, help your body fight off viruses, bacteria, and toxins.

Raw milk contains a broad selection of vitamins and minerals, ranging from calcium and phosphorus, to vitamins A and D, and magnesium, in perfect balance. Raw grass-fed dairy also contains a nutrient missing from our diets, called vitamin K2, which is extremely valuable in helping the body absorb calcium, and therefore rebuilding bone, repairing cavities, and keeping the blood vessels clear of calcium deposits. Only grass-fed milk, cheese and butter contains this important nutrient.

There are more than 60 functioning enzymes in raw milk that perform amazing work. These enzymes in milk assist in the digestion process and help the body break down and use all the healthy nutrients that milk contains. Amylase, lactase, lipase and phosphatase in raw milk break down starch, lactose, fat and phosphate compounds, making milk more easily digestible. Other enzymes, like catalase, lysozyme, and lactoperoxidase help to protect milk from unwanted bacterial infections, making raw milk safe to drink.

What about the safety of raw milk? We have all been lead to believe that milk MUST be pasteurized to kill bacteria and unwanted dangerous pathogens. But milk straight from a healthy cow's udder is actually very clean. And a cow fed a natural diet and not pumped full of hormones and antibiotics is naturally a healthier cow, free from infections and an irritated udder.

Why pasteurize milk then? Pasteurization began in the early 1900's when dairy production increased and unsanitary milking conditions were causing illness. Sickly dairy cows, dirty conditions and unsanitary milking procedures are more likely the cause of bacteria in raw milk. Pasteurized milk actually has sickened thousands of people, even more than the reports of raw milk making people sick. The dairy industry and the huge industrialized dairy farms have fought to have raw milk made illegal, and many states now make it hard to obtain raw milk.

But while raw milk has valuable enzymes in it that actually kill off pathogens, these beneficial enzymes are destroyed by pasteurization. Consequently, there are no remaining safety systems left when harmful bacteria get into the pasteurized milk. What about the stories of people getting sick from raw milk? These stories have proven to be not directly connected to the milk, but to other unsanitary conditions unassociated with the milk.

What about cholesterol? Raw dairy contains a decent amount of cholesterol—about 3mg of cholesterol per gram. Our bodies make most of the cholesterol we need. The amount will fluctuate however, depending on what we get from food. Cholesterol in and of itself is not a harmful product as it is a protective/repair substance our body uses as a building block for a number of key hormones, or as a repair material. It's natural, normal, and essential, and it's found in our brain, liver, nerves, blood, bile, and every cell membrane.

One important item to note about raw, fresh milk—the taste! You have never tasted milk this delicious from a grocery store. Wow! Nothing tastes better. From the first sip, you will be hooked, even if you were not a big milk-drinker before. There is absolutely no comparison between fresh raw milk, and thin pasteurized processed stuff you get from the grocery store.

Know the source of your raw milk and demand that it be from well-kept, grass-fed animals. Preferably organic. Raw milk is harder to find, as many states will not allow it to be sold commercially, but you can look up the closest source of raw milk to where you live on this website: http://www.realmilk.com

My recommendation is to avoid milk altogether unless you can find a co-op or quality farm that sells raw milk from grass-fed cows. RealMilk.com is a great place to find co-ops and farms that sell raw milk in your area. I was surprised to find multiple places in different areas that I've lived over the years where I could buy healthy raw milk for my family.

These farms also delivered some of the highest quality eggs, yogurt, grass-fed meats, and raw cheeses I've ever seen as well. If you get hooked up with a great farm, you can easily reduce your dependence by 50% on the low quality junk that most grocery stores sell you. Even in major cities, I've been able to find farms or co-ops that deliver to the cities. So, do a little research, and you may be able to greatly improve your family's food quality.

By the way, if you're still "afraid" of raw milk, even after reading this, your fears are unfounded. My family and I have drunk hundreds of gallons of raw milk for almost 10 years now and nobody has ever gotten sick from it. In contrast to the unsanitary conditions of most commercial dairy farms (and the poor health of their cows which increases the risk of pathogens being present in the milk), most raw milk farms are some of the cleanest dairy operations around with some of the healthiest cows too.

CHAPTER 15
The Healthiest Fats—Surprising Information

I am a strong proponent of including a variety of healthy oils and fats into your diet. Together they work as a team to supply your body with essential fatty acids for longevity, hormone balance, heart health, sharp vision, glowing moist skin and energy. The wonderful variety of oils and fats certainly includes organic, preferably grass-fed butter, lard, coconut oil, and extra virgin olive oil.

Twenty five years ago or so, everyone switched from natural fat sources like butter and lard, to processed margarine and Crisco, because the medical community decided that butter, lard and other saturated fats caused heart disease, heart attacks and strokes. What happened? Even though today we eat far less butter and lard than we did at the turn of the century, heart disease has skyrocketed! Clearly this isn't the answer.

It is not the cholesterol and saturated fats in our diets that contributes to heart attacks, but a combination of high blood sugar from too much sugary, starchy foods, and eating highly processed vegetable oils high in inflammatory omega 6 fats, including soybean oil, sunflower oil, corn oil, safflower oil and canola oil. These foods increase the inflammation in blood vessels. This irritation in blood vessels causes the cholesterol buildup that is characteristic of heart disease.

Long ago, households cooked with lard, a natural animal fat. But then along came hydrogenated vegetable oil (Crisco) that was supposedly better for you. As we mentioned before, this trans fat is extremely toxic to the body and should be avoided at all costs.

In contrast, lard looks like a much healthier choice. Lard's fat is also mostly monounsaturated fat. And, the saturated fat in lard really has no effect on blood cholesterol. Lard has a higher smoking point than other fats, allowing foods that you cook in it to absorb less grease. It does not produce toxic by-products like vegetable oils when exposed to high heat, rather it remains stable. The best type of lard or beef tallow should come from grass-fed animals because they contain the higher quantities of the omega 3 fats and CLA.

Of course, natural fats in general are beneficial to the body. Fat is converted to fuel, which is burned as an energy source, as long as you are not eating a diet high in sugar or starch. Fat helps our bodies absorb nutrients, particularly calcium and fat-soluble vitamins A, D, E and K. People who eat diet rich in natural fats like lard, butter and coconut oil, along with healthy omega 3 fats will have far less wrinkles in their skin than people who eat a diet that consists mostly of vegetable oils.

Many endurance athletes are now turning to healthy fats as a form of high performance fuel which provides a better and more long lasting supply of energy than sugary gels, Gu's and energy drinks.

Butter or Margarine?

Most margarines are pure junk that should never be consumed by humans. Despite the propaganda that you've been fed by the crooked marketing tactics of food manufacturing companies over the years, margarine is not healthier than butter!

In fact, since margarine is a often a major source of harmful artificial trans fats, produced by highly refined inflammatory vegetable oils, high temperature, high pressure, and petroleum solvents—margarine is more closely related to a inedible industrial oil rather than something that should be thought of as food—even those so-called 'healthy spreads.'

Don't believe it!

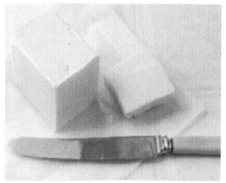

Butter, on the other hand, is a natural food that has been around since our ancestors first started domesticating animals. Butter has been used for around 4500 years!

Butter is a completely natural food that is essential to your health, especially when you eat organic, grass-fed butter. It is high in vitamins, minerals and other power-packed nutrients. Look at some of the other benefits of REAL grass-fed butter:

- Butter contains conjugated linoleic acid, (CLA), a powerful fat burner, muscle builder, anti-cancer agent, and immunity booster.

- Butterfat is a source of quick energy, and also a great endurance energy source.

- Butter contains the essential fatty acid, Arachidonic Acid which is an important muscle building and fat burning compound.

- Butter is a great source of vitamins A. Butter contains the most easily absorbable form of vitamin A, which among other things is good for the skin, the eyes, the thyroid, and the adrenal glands.

- Grass-fed butter is one of the very few foods that contain vitamin K2, found only in the milk of grass-fed animals. It is necessary to get calcium in the bones and teeth.

- Butter contains high levels of vitamin D, also essential to absorption of calcium, strengthening the immune system and overall feelings of well-being.

- Butter contains the vital mineral selenium, which is a powerful cancer-fighting nutrient.

- Butter contains iodine in highly absorbable form—highly recommended for proper thyroid function and fat metabolism.

- Butter is a good source of lauric acid, important for your immune system, and also in fighting fungal infections.

- Butter actually protects against tooth decay.

- Butter contains lecithin, which is essential for healthy brain function and cholesterol metabolism.

- Butter fights free radical damage with its antioxidants.

The bottom line is that if you're deciding whether to use butter or margarine, you're ALWAYS better off using butter, as it is a real food with real benefits compared to the "fake food" margarine. Keep in mind that butter still is a highly concentrated source of calories, so be aware of controlling your portion sizes. However, since butter gives you some very important and necessary nutrition that your body needs, it will reduce appetite and cravings.

Similar to what we've discussed regarding other dairy products, the only source of healthy butter is from grass-fed cows. Once again, www.RealMilk. com can help you to find sources of raw grass-fed dairy products near you. If you can't find butter from grass-fed cows, your next best bet is to look for organic or grass-fed at your health food store or your grocery store.

Coconut Oil – A Healthy Saturated Fat?

Coconut oil is preferred by athletes, body builders and those on diets. The reason is because coconut oil is made up unique healthy saturated fats called medium chain triglycerides (MCTs) which are quickly converted into energy. Coconut oil boosts energy and endurance, and enhances the athletic performance.

Coconut oil is one of the best body fat burning fuels you can find. When you eat coconut oil (I like it in my smoothies), it is immediately processed as fuel for energy, unlike other fats that require a longer process.

The short and medium-chain fatty acids rev up the body's metabolism, and keep your energy going for a long time, without the crash that sugary carbohydrates can have. It is also easy to digest and aids the healthy functioning of the thyroid gland (critical to metabolism and weight loss) and enzyme systems.

People who live in tropical coastal areas and eat coconut oil daily and use it as a primary cooking oil, are normally not overweight. Pure coconut oil (make sure it is not hydrogenated) is actually one of the best options for cooking oil, due to its highly stable nature under heat. This makes it much less inflammatory to your body compared to other oils such as soybean oil, corn oil, or other "vegetable" oils. This article below describes more details about cooking oils and which are healthy vs. unhealthy: http://www.truthaboutabs.com/ unhealthy-vs-healthy-cooking-oils.html

Fats have come full circle; we are now reverting back to the good traditional fats that our ancestors have cooked with for years. Long before heart disease, cancer and other serious diseases made their appearance, these fats were used in abundance. Now we are beginning to realize they are not the villains they have been made out to be. So enjoy your butter, coconut oil and lard, and feel good about it!

Maximize Your Flat Belly Journey: Get Powerful Fat Loss Secrets From Key Food And Fitness Experts.
http://velocityhousepresents.com/FlatBellyKitchen

By Mike Geary, Certified Personal Trainer, Certified Nutrition Specialist
& Catherine Ebeling – RN, BSN

CHAPTER 16
Nuts About Nuts

A high-fat food that helps you lose weight? If you have read the previous chapters, you may start to see a message here. Yes! Certain high fat foods are actually fat burning and belly flattening, and nuts are definitely one of them! Forget about shying away from nuts and put them at the top of your list of healthy lean-body snacks!

Almonds and walnuts sit at the top of the list for nutrition, but many other varieties of nuts are healthy, too, including pistachios, pecans, cashews, macadamias, brazil nuts, and even (the legumes) peanuts. Numerous studies have shown that dieters who include nuts in their diet actually lose more weight than those who avoid nuts. Nuts are the perfect snack.

As long as you can restrain yourself from whole bags at a time, nuts can actually be fat-fighters and help with weight loss. Protein and fat in nuts helps you feel satisfied and stop cravings, and since nuts have no sugars, they keep your blood sugar stable, in the fat burning zone, which means they are more likely to be used as energy. Nuts will not put you on that merry-go-round of eating, hunger, more eating, and weight gain, like carbs do.

Besides their lean body benefits, nuts are a highly nutritious food to include in your diet. Most nuts are high in monounsaturated fats, the same type of health-promoting fats as are found in olive oil, which have been associated with reduced risk of heart disease and cancer. Nuts also contain polyunsaturated fats, healthy saturated fats, and linoleic acid, another healthy fat that the body utilizes for essential fatty acids. Eating healthy fats can satisfy your cravings and keep you from over-indulging in something like cookies, cake or chips.

Nuts have loads of great nutrition, although their fat content (75 to 95 percent of total calories) means you shouldn't eat them by the bucket. But because they are so satisfying to your appetite, you probably won't need to eat too many. Macadamia, the gourmet of nuts, is the highest in fat (but still healthy fats). Macadamia nuts are one of the only food sources that contain palmitoleic acid (a type of monounsaturated fatty acid that helps speed up fat metabolism, reducing the body's ability to store fat). Walnuts, Brazil nuts and pine nuts are extra rich in omega 3 fatty acids, and Brazil nuts have exceptionally high levels of the mineral selenium which has some very powerful antioxidant properties and protects cells from free radical damage, while helping you burn fat better.

Although technically, peanuts are a legume (like beans), they provide the most complete protein. Many other nuts are missing the amino acid lysine, but peanuts contain all the essential amino acids. Peanuts are also rich in antioxidant polyphenols like those found in berries.

Five significant human research studies all found that nut consumption is linked to a lower risk for heart disease. Researchers who studied data from the Nurses' Health Study estimated that substituting nuts for an equivalent amount of carbohydrate in an average diet resulted in a 30% reduction in heart disease risk. Nuts contain significant amounts of vitamin E. As an antioxidant, vitamin E can help prevent the oxidation of LDL cholesterol, which can damage arteries.

Nuts are chock-full of hard-to-get minerals, such as copper, iron, magnesium, manganese, zinc and selenium. Iron helps your blood deliver oxygen to your muscles and brain, while zinc helps boost your immune system and healthy brain function. Selenium is a potent cancer-fighting mineral, and aids the thyroid gland, which regulates metabolism and fat-burning in the body.

Potassium is an important electrolyte involved in nerve transmission, heart function and blood pressure. Nuts are good for your cardiovascular health by providing 257 mg of potassium and only trace amounts of sodium (that's if you eat the unsalted kind!), making them an especially good choice in protecting against high blood pressure and atherosclerosis.

Magnesium is nature's calming agent. When your body has enough magnesium, veins and arteries relax and dilate, which lowers blood pressure and improves the flow of blood, oxygen and nutrients throughout the body. This mineral is also relaxing mentally as well as physically. Magnesium is essential for prevention of heart attacks.

Nuts are also a good source of fiber and protein, which of course, you know helps to control blood sugar and can aid in weight loss. While all nuts are healthy, there a few superstars:

By Mike Geary, Certified Personal Trainer, Certified Nutrition Specialist
& Catherine Ebeling – RN, BSN

Brazil nuts contain a very high amount of selenium: about 70 to 90 micrograms per nut. So only 3-4 Brazil nuts will provide you with ample amounts of this essential nutrient. And, nuts do their part to keep bones strong by providing magnesium, manganese, and boron, essential for bone health.

A serving of almonds contains almost 99 mg of magnesium (that's 25% of the daily value for this important mineral), plus 257 mg of potassium, in addition to healthy fats and vitamin E.

Walnuts, pecans, and chestnuts have the highest antioxidant content of the tree nuts, with walnuts winning out over the others in antioxidant content. And, peanuts also contribute significantly to our dietary intake of antioxidants.

Pistachios help to reduce the risk of macular degeneration, a common cause of visual loss in older individuals. Pistachios contain two important carotenoids, lutein and zeaxanthin, compounds which help prevent this common eye condition. Carotenoids are strong antioxidants that help to offset cell injury and damage. A daily snack of pistachios could be a tasty and effective way to protect one of your most important senses—your vision. Pistachios are also high in protein, making a satisfying snack.

The list of health benefits attached to each individual nut is endless. Other nuts that are particularly good include: pecans for prostate health, hazelnuts for their large amounts of vitamin E, and cashews for their iron content. Choose raw nuts or raw nut butters instead of roasted nuts if you can; it helps to maintain the quality and nutritional content of the healthy fats that you will eat.

Remember that polyunsaturated fats are unstable and become inflammatory to your body when they've been exposed to heat, so roasted nuts are not the best option. Stay away from the commercially prepared roasted and salted nuts, as these often have undesirable cottonseed or soybean oils added, thus canceling out the many of the healthy effects of the nuts.

And for an added change, try almond butter, cashew butter, pecan butter, or macadamia butter to add variety to your diet and make it easier to get more of the quality nutrition of nuts into your diet.

CHAPTER 17
Avocados

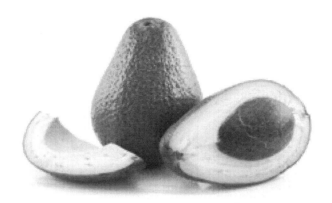

Avocados are another so-called "fatty food" that many of us have been conditioned to avoid, but this is a power-packed super food! Not only is this fruit super high in monounsaturated fat, but also chock full of vitamins, minerals, micronutrients, and antioxidants.

The healthy fats and other nutrition you get from avocados help your body to stabilize blood sugar and insulin, which helps with fat loss and muscle building. The healthy fat content in avocados makes you feel full longer and takes away junk food cravings. And that equals a leaner, healthier body.

Avocados contain plenty of oleic acid, the same monounsaturated fat in olive oil, which helps lower cholesterol and is helpful in preventing breast cancer and other cancers. Avocados are also a good source of potassium, a mineral that helps regulate blood pressure and electrolytes. Adequate intake of potassium can help to guard against circulatory diseases, like high blood pressure, heart disease, or stroke.

One cup of avocado has about a quarter of your required daily amount of folate, or folic acid, a B vitamin that plays an essential role in making new cells by helping to produce healthy DNA and RNA. Folate is required for pregnant women, and helps lower the risk birth defects in babies, as well as being important for heart health. One study showed that individuals who consume folate-rich diets have a much lower risk of cardiovascular disease or stroke than those who do not consume as much of this vital nutrient.

Avocados are also a very concentrated dietary source of the carotenoid, lutein which is good for eye health. It also contains measurable amounts of related carotenoids, zeaxanthin, alpha-carotene and beta-carotene, plus significant quantities of vitamin E, all significant cancer-fighting ingredients.

Since avocados contain a large variety of nutrients including vitamins, minerals, as well as healthy fat, enjoying a few slices of avocado in your tossed salad, or mixing some chopped avocado into your favorite salsa will not only add a rich, creamy flavor, but will actually increase your body's ability to absorb the healthy nutrients in your salad.

Cut up fresh avocados in your salad; add to sandwiches, omelets, or Mexican food. Eat it right out of the shell with a spoon and a squeeze of lime, or mix up a little guacamole (mashed avocados with garlic, onion, tomato, pepper, lemon juice) for a super delicious and nutritious satisfying snack. Avoid the fattening corn chips and dip veggies in your guacamole instead, or eat with a fork, or spread on a juicy grass-fed hamburger. There are a zillion delicious ways to enjoy avocados! Avocados are best when firm but yield slightly to touch.

CHAPTER 18
Berries and Super Fruits

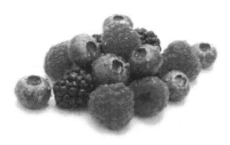

Berries—including blueberries, strawberries, raspberries, and even the "exotic" Goji berry, and acai berry are powerhouses of nutrition, packed with vitamins and minerals, and also some of the best sources of antioxidants of any food in existence! Berries also contain a healthy dose of fiber, which slows your carbohydrate absorption and digestion, and controls blood sugar levels to help prevent insulin spikes, making berries a great superfood for fat loss and a lean body!

Include the familiar berries as well as some of the more exotic berries: blueberries, strawberries, blackberries, raspberries, and the rare Goji berries (which are one of the most nutrient-dense, highest antioxidant berries on earth), or the spectacular Acai berries.

A cup of strawberries contains over 100 mg of vitamin C, which is better than orange juice. Vitamin C strengthens the immune system and helps build strong connective tissue. Strawberries contain calcium, magnesium, folate and potassium and very few calories. If they are available, organic strawberries are better tasting than conventional and well worth the extra price.

Non-organic strawberries are one of the highest sprayed crops and since strawberries really have no skin or rind, they soak up all those pesticides and herbicides. Even washing won't get rid of that.

One cup of blueberries offers a smaller amount of vitamin C, but high amounts of minerals and phytochemicals and very low calories. Blueberries are also extremely high in antioxidants, as are cranberries. And raspberries offer vitamin C and potassium and a variety of other antioxidants. You can choose other berries with similar power-packed nutrition, such as loganberries, currants, gooseberries, lingonberries and bilberries.

The pigments in berries that create the bright colors are also good for your health. Berries contain potent phytochemicals and flavonoids that may help to prevent cancer, reduce heart disease risk, and protect skin from damage. Blueberries and raspberries also contain lutein, which is important for healthy vision.

Every grocery store carries a wide variety of fresh and frozen berries. Look for ripe, colorful and firm berries with no sign of mold or mushy spots. Berries are also found in the frozen section of the grocery store. Once they thaw, they will not be as firm as freshly picked berries, but they are still delicious and good for you. Throwing them into the blender for a smoothie is a great way to enjoy frozen berries in the winter.

For the freshest berries, try farmers' markets that offer local berries harvested that same day. Some berry farms allow you to pick your own berries. Nothing is better than picking and eating berries warm from the sun and bursting with freshness and nutrients!

Berry Smoothie

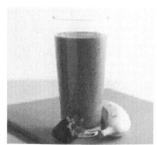

My very favorite easy berry smoothie can be made with a cup or so of frozen berries, 1 banana, a scoop of your favorite protein powder (or if you don't have protein powder, throw in a raw, free range, organic egg—it's perfect protein), a half cup of orange juice or any other juice you have, a few ice cubes, and blend. These are delicious and nutritious and the protein makes them a satisfying meal or snack. And don't worry about the raw egg—raw eggs are fine as long as the shell is intact. And if you're using fresh farm eggs instead of the grocery store kind, they are even safer. Rinse them off before using.

CHAPTER 19
Leafy, Green, and Gorgeous

Did you know our ancient ancestors used to eat up to six pounds of leafy greens a day? As they walked from place to place, they picked and ate green leaves as they went. That's a lot of greens! Very few of us even get the minimum of three cups a week! Yet, these leafy greens deliver a bonanza of fat burning nutrition like vitamins, minerals, fiber, antioxidants, and phytonutrients!

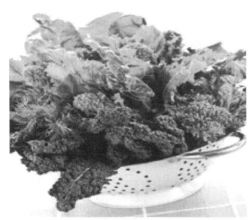

Leafy vegetables are the ideal flat belly food, as they are typically very low in calories. They are useful in reducing the risk of cancer and heart disease since they are low in fat, high in dietary fiber, and rich in folic acid, vitamins K, C, E, and many of the B vitamins, iron, calcium, potassium and magnesium, as well as containing a host of powerful phytochemicals.

Did you know that eating 3 or more servings a week of green leafy vegetables significantly reduces the risk of stomach cancer, the fourth most frequent cancer in the world? Cruciferous vegetables like cabbage, cauliflower, Brussels sprouts, and broccoli are rich in natural chemicals called indoles and isothiocyanates, which protect against colon cancer, and other cancers. And broccoli sprouts contain 10 times as much sulforaphane, a cancer-protective substance, than mature broccoli.

Dark green leafy vegetables are, for a low calorie food, one of the most concentrated sources of nutrition of any food. They also provide a variety of phytonutrients including beta-carotene, lutein, and zeaxanthin, which protect all of our cells from damage and our eyes from macular degeneration and cataracts, among other benefits. Dark green leaves even contain small amounts of healthy omega 3 fats.

The rock star nutrient in greens is vitamin K. A cup of most cooked greens provides at least nine times the minimum recommended intake of vitamin K, and even a couple of cups of dark green leafy salad greens will give you the minimum all on their own. Recent research has provided evidence that this vitamin may be even more important than we once thought and many people do not get nearly enough of it.

Some of the fantastic benefits of Vitamin K:

- Regulates blood clotting

- May help prevent and possibly even reduce atherosclerosis by reducing calcium in arterial plaques.

- A key regulator of inflammation, and helps protect us from inflammatory diseases including arthritis.

- Vitamin K is a fat-soluble vitamin, so make sure to use a dressing with healthy fats (such as extra virgin olive oil or Udo's choice Oil blend) on your salad, or add avocado slices to your salad. Adding a small amount of butter or cheese to cooked veggies can also help with vitamin absorption.

Here's an article that gives ideas for making your own super-healthy salad dressings and avoiding the junk that's in most store bought dressings:

Greens have very few carbohydrates in them, and lots of fiber, which make them slower to digest. So, greens have very little impact on blood sugar. In some diets, greens are even treated as a "freebie" carb-wise (meaning the carbohydrate doesn't have to be counted). All of which means—lean, mean nutrition! I think of greens as being in three different groups, depending on how you prepare them:

Salad greens—Usually best eaten raw. Follow this key rule when selecting salad greens: the darker the color, the more nutritious. Iceberg lettuce, for example, is extremely low in nutrients, and is virtually worthless nutritionally. Lettuce's more colorful family members are much more worthy of attention. For example, romaine lettuce, red leaf lettuce, bib lettuce, and baby greens have 8 times the vitamin A, and 6 times the vitamin C as iceberg lettuce. Bib lettuce, and red and green leaf lettuce make great substitutes for bread too. Try a tuna salad wrapped in lettuce instead of bread, or any of your other favorite sandwiches, it's a better, lower carb, grain free option!

When you have a choice, a variety of greens is always best, as each has its own family of nutrients. Go for as many different colors and shades of green as you can! One of the best choices is baby greens. These tender leaves usually come in a wide variety of greens, each with their own treasure trove of nutrients, and what's more, they are delicious!

Green, leafy vegetables provide a great variety of colors from the dark bluish-green of kale to the bright spring green of romaine lettuce.
Leafy greens run the whole gamut of flavors, from sweet and nutty to bitter, peppery, or earthy. Young plants generally have small, tender leaves and a mild flavor. Many mature plants have tougher leaves and stronger flavors.

Two of my favorites are mache and baby arugula. Arugula has been one of my favorite healthy additions recently to top grass-fed burgers or added to the side of omelets. Arugula has a super-high nutrient density and a delicious nutty, spicy flavor!

Quick-cooking Greens—can either be eaten raw or lightly cooked. Spinach is the best-known example in this category. It takes only seconds to cook a spinach leaf. And overcooked spinach is not very tasty. Cooked greens shrink quickly so you can get lots of concentrated nutrition from them. Six cups of raw greens become approximately one cup of cooked greens.

Most quick-cooking greens take just a few minutes to cook—and should not be overcooked or they become mushy and tasteless. Swiss chard is a quick-cooking green, and also can be eaten raw, though it isn't usually. Chard is now available in many colors, which are often milder-tasting than the more traditional chard. I recently saw a suggestion to chop up the stems and put them in tuna salad instead of celery. If you haven't tried chard, you really should—you may be surprised! Chard and the more familiar spinach are good places to start with cooked greens, as they are so easy, and not as bitter as some others. Beet greens are also quick cooking (and delicious), and are actually related to chard and spinach. Escarole, dandelion greens, and sorrel are also relatively quick-cooking greens.

Hearty Greens—many people seem to have a deep-seated fear and dislike of kale and collard greens (at least outside the southern U.S.), but I encourage you to give them a try, as they have the most nutritional benefits of all. Over time, they may even become favorites.

Kale and collard greens are the most common examples of hearty greens. They do require cooking, although not as much as many people think. Yes, you can cook collards for an hour, but if you cut the greens from the fibrous stems they can be tender in 10-15 minutes.

How to Cook Greens

Greens can be braised (cooked fairly slowly in a small amount of liquid, usually a flavorful stock), sautéed (cooked quickly in a small amount of oil), or a combination of the two. They can also be steamed or boiled, and taste especially good with chopped fresh garlic, small bits of cooked bacon, lemon, vinegar, hot chilies, anchovies, or onion. Just remember that greens taste best when they are very lightly cooked. Take them off the heat when they are just limp but still bright green. Throw greens into almost any soup or skillet dish, or even omelets, especially the milder-tasting greens such as chard.

CHAPTER 20
Sweetness! Stevia, Real Maple Syrup, Raw Honey

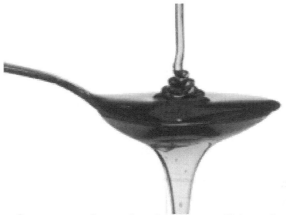

Our craving for sweets often ruins the most well intentioned flat belly body plan, and we succumb to that candy bar, a handful of cookies, a slice of cake, a generous scoop of ice cream, or other such decadent fare. The key ingredient in all of these items and essentially most of the sweets available on the market is sugar or high fructose corn syrup.

Too much sugar is often the culprit in sabotaging our diets, and making us gain weight, but it seems hard to avoid or resist. Sometimes you just crave a little something sweet. 'Diet' treats are even worse, because they usually contain artificial sweeteners, chemical flavorings and more things that will just cause weight gain. Fortunately a variety of natural sweeteners that are quite common in supermarkets, may be sitting on your shelf in your pantry at this very moment.

Honey is an excellent alternative to sugar and has some healthy benefits for you compared to refined white sugar. Although honey is still a form of sugar (and you need to be aware of its caloric impact), one benefit of honey vs. refined sugar is that several studies have found that raw honey can actually improve your body's ability to process glucose. On the other hand, refined sugar negatively affects your body's ability to process glucose over time.

Different types of honey contain different nutrients and health benefits, depending on the types of pollen and flowers the honey comes from. All honey

Maximize Your Flat Belly Journey: Get Powerful Fat Loss Secrets From Key Food And Fitness Experts.
http://velocityhousepresents.com/FlatBellyKitchen

possesses antibacterial agents and acts as an antioxidant. Honey contains vitamins B2 and B6, and is a good source of iron. Consuming just a spoonful of honey each day can raise the antioxidant levels in our bodies, and it is also a healthier natural sweetener available for those with Type 2 Diabetes. Raw honey, which is chock full of valuable enzymes, can often be found at Whole Foods, Trader Joe's, local farm stands, and even some grocery stores or health food stores, and is by far the best kind of honey you can get.

Honey is a great replacement for sugar in many recipes, and because it is quite a bit sweeter, you can use a smaller amount. The rule of thumb is about a 1/2-cup of honey per cup of sugar. Also when cooking, you should also reduce liquids in the recipe by a 1/4 cup to ensure proper consistency. Honey also serves to brown foods more easily as they cook, so lower cooking temperatures 25 degrees F.

Real maple syrup is another product many of us may have in our homes and another natural sweetener that can often be used in place of sugar. We are talking about real, pure, natural maple syrup—NOT the maple flavored corn syrup! Real maple syrup is a good source of minerals and trace nutrients. As with honey, maple syrup is also a useful antioxidant, and possesses a good amount of zinc, which can help prevent atherosclerosis and lower cholesterol, as well as strengthen the immune system.

Maple syrup can be purchased in three specific colors or grades, each having a particular flavor. The lighter syrups (grade A) will possess a more subtle flavor, while the darkest syrup (grade B or C) yields the strongest, sweetest flavor. The darker maple syrups typically contain higher antioxidant and nutrient levels than Grade A maple syrup.

As with honey, you need to be aware of the calories maple syrup contains, and the effect it has on blood sugar, but it is definitely a better choice than refined white sugar. My personal preference is to use just a tiny drizzle of real maple syrup in coffee instead of white sugar. For teas, I like a small dab of raw honey instead of refined sugar. Maple syrup is also great on oatmeal too along with some grass-fed butter.

Even though honey and maple syrup are healthier options compared to refined white sugar, your best bet is to reduce your dependence on sweeteners by learning to train your taste buds to prefer less sweetness. I have trained my taste buds to prefer the taste of unsweetened iced tea, compared to years ago when I absolutely had to have some sweetener. Same with coffee – although I still occasionally use a small dab of real maple syrup in my coffee, I've adapted my taste buds to be able to enjoy plain black coffee as well.

Blackstrap molasses is another option for a natural sweetener used in baking. Blackstrap molasses is rich in iron and B vitamins, manganese, calcium, potassium, and more. It is less sweet and lower in calories than other natural sweeteners.

Because molasses has such a strong and distinctive flavor, you may not want to use it as often to replace sugar, but it can give some foods a unique flavor, such as baked beans and gingerbread.

Stevia, a better natural sweetener option that is calorie-free

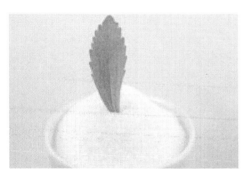

Although Stevia has been around for years, it is just now showing up as a sweetener in the United States. Stevia comes from the leaves of a shrub native to Paraguay and Brazil, and has been used as a sweetener for many years in South America. Stevia has been used for several decades in Japan with no negative health effects.

Stevia is about three hundred times sweeter than sugar, and has all the benefits of a sweetener without being bad for you or fattening. It's truly natural, not some scary chemical compound from a laboratory, it's free of calories, doesn't promote tooth decay, and won't elevate blood sugar levels or cause weight gain.

To sugar-crazy and diet-conscious Americans, stevia should be incredibly popular and well known, but up until recently, it was not allowed in foods or easily found. The Food and Drug Administration (FDA) banned stevia in 1991. Why?

Maximize Your Flat Belly Journey: Get Powerful Fat Loss Secrets From Key Food And Fitness Experts.
http://velocityhousepresents.com/FlatBellyKitchen

Like many proponents of stevia, the sugar industry was involved in this. The FDA ban allowed it to only be sold as a dietary 'supplement', and it can be found in most health food stores in the supplement aisle, right next to the vitamins. It was difficult to find and never in the sugar or sweetener aisle, until lately.

However, stevia is becoming much more popular and is showing up in a lot of foods and beverages lately. You may see food items now sweetened with Truvia.

Stevia is the standout sweetener in the marketplace, because it is what the public is looking for in a low-calorie sweetener to replace the questionable and unnatural Sweet n' Low, Splenda, and NutraSweet chemical artificial sweeteners.

Stevia's sweetness comes from its leaves. The stevia leaves are milled, and a freshwater brewing method is used to extract the sweetness. This extract is then purified further until a very high purity Reb-A is obtained.

While the previous chemically-processed artificial sweeteners have been connected to lung tumors, breast tumors, and other rare types of tumors; several forms of leukemia, and chronic respiratory disease in several rodent studies, as well as rashes, headaches, neurological problems, and other serious and nasty side effects, stevia, Reb-A and its derivatives seem to be the safest of all low-calorie sweeteners for the moment.

You can find stevia blends for your own use at this site:
http://www.Naturally-Stevia.com

Try Stevia in your favorite beverages like coffee, tea, lemonade, and more. Depending on the brand and type of Stevia you use, the taste may vary. Now that Stevia is becoming more mainstream, the taste has improved. And some Stevia comes in a liquid form with great flavors like vanilla, toffee, black cherry, lemon, etc. Give it a try!

CHAPTER 21
REAL Energy in a Bar

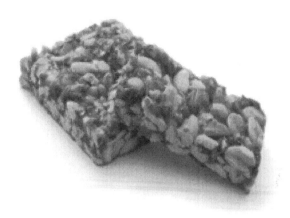

Whether out on a mega-mile bike ride, running, or just on the run, occasionally you need to have something on hand for a quick and healthy snack. While "energy bars" are marketed this way, many are deceiving in that they are actually just glorified candy bars full of sugar, corn syrup and artificial ingredients—nothing our bodies really need—especially if we want them to be lean, healthy, and strong.

However, there actually are a few really good energy bars out there. They may not be as easy to find, but when you do find them, these bars are worth keeping around. When looking for a healthy energy bar, look for a short list of natural ingredients (that you recognize), little sugar, and a genuine protein source like whey or nuts, as opposed to soy protein. This is what I have found so far:

- **Organic Food Bars**—This is actually the brand name.
  Depending on which flavor, these are usually a base of organic almond or cashew butter, with a certain type of fruit, organic seeds, organic bio-sprouts (quinoa, etc), and some organic rice protein. Some flavors include an organic dark chocolate as well. They also have a line of bars that use exclusively raw ingredients.

Not only are these food bars extremely nutritious, but I think they are delicious as well and offer a lot of flavors to choose from: blueberry, cranberry, chocolate chip, high protein, and more.

- **Dale's Raw Food bars** -These taste great and include these great flavors:

  -Blueberry Macadamia
  -Strawberry Banana
  -Raspberry Hazelnut
  -Chocolate Chia Maca
  -and Low-Carb Cafe Mocha

  Just remember that we weren't big fans of the "Goji and greens" flavor...
  But the other five that I listed above we really loved!

  You can grab some of these tasty Raw Protein bars here.

- **Kind Fruit and Nut Bars** – These bars are one of my favorites and seem to be showing up everywhere now. These bars are made up of primarily nuts and dried fruits, although there are many new flavors appearing as well, like peanut butter and dark chocolate with protein, and dark chocolate cherry cashew. Kind bars are natural bars made from wholesome ingredients you can see and pronounce. They are gluten-free, soy free, dairy free and corn free and contain just the right mix of nuts for protein and healthy fats, along with a touch of sweetness from the dried fruits.

- **Larabars**—These are even simpler in ingredients than the Organic food bars. Larabar is a delicious blend of unsweetened fruits, nuts and spices—energy in its purest form. Made from 100% whole food, each flavor contains no more than eight ingredients, but most flavors only have 2 to 3 ingredients. Sweet with no added sweeteners, except for dates. Sustaining with no added fillers, supplements or flavorings. Just real, whole food loaded with nature's own minerals and vitamins. All of the vitamins, minerals, fiber, protein, good carbohydrates and healthy fats are uncooked and unprocessed. They are gluten-free, dairy free, soy free, vegan, and kosher. Some of the flavors are: coconut cream pie, chocolate mole, chocolate coconut, cherry pie, apple pie, ginger snap and more.

The essential enzymes, which are necessary for the digestion and utilization of nutrients, remain completely intact in their most natural effective state. A diet abundant in raw, unprocessed foods is important for health and longevity.

- **Prograde Cravers**—These are made by Prograde Nutrition. These are definitely some of the tastiest nutrition bars I've ever had (especially the peanut butter flavor!) and they are also made with all organic ingredients using nut butters, rice protein, organic dark chocolate, etc. These are not really that high in protein and are more of an organic snack bar. These aren't available in stores and you can only find these organic bars online at: http://natural.getprograde.com/cravers

- **Boomi Bar** – These bars are sweetened with honey, all natural, and contain primarily nuts and fruit. There are several different, delicious flavors to choose from. For example, the Macadamia Paradise bar contains: macadamia nuts, pineapple, honey, raisin, sesame seeds, puffed amaranth, crisped rice and salt.

- **Go Raw Bars** – Another favorite is Go Raw bars. These are just what they say, made of organic, raw, dehydrated ingredients. They generally have only a few ingredients and they are simple, delicious and very healthy. My personal favorite is the Live Pumpkin bar. It contains sprouted organic pumpkin seeds, sprouted flax seeds, dates, agave nectar, and sea salt. There are other great flavors, like Banana Bread Flax, Spirulina, Live Granola, and Real Live Apricot. These bars are gluten-free, corn and soy free, and for those of you who may be allergic to nuts, these bars are nut free as well.

When you actually find truly healthy nutrition bars like these examples above, they make great quick snacks while you're traveling or while you're at work or just need a quick pick-me-up energy bar at any time.

Carry some with you or in your car, just to make sure there are healthy options to choose when you are ravenous—that way you won't be as tempted by fast food joints or junk food vending machines.

Stores like Whole Foods have other whole, raw healthy energy bars as well, like Jay Robb Bars, Perfect Food Bars, Greens Plus Omega 3, Chia Bars, Bliss bars and others. Even some grocery stores are beginning to carry wider choices.

Just be sure to avoid processed ingredients like refined flours, soy protein, and a lot of sugars, and choose the bars with easily identifiable and NATURAL ingredients. Just be aware that at typical chain grocery stores, mega-stores like Wal-Mart and most convenient stores, 99% of the bars they have are usually made with soy protein, chemical additives, and loads of sweeteners.

CHAPTER 22
A Dark and Mysterious Treat

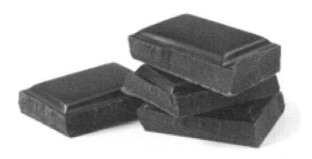

Every once in a while you need a sweet, satisfying treat, and chocolate seems to fit the bill. Chocolate is actually good for you, but it can't be just any old chocolate you grab off the shelf. I am certainly not talking about M&M's or a big ol' Hershey bar! That's just cheap chocolate with lower levels of actual cocoa and lots of refined sugar and other junk.

One of the major reasons diets and other weight loss programs fail is because you end up feeling deprived. Life isn't about that. It's about changing your bad habits, and allowing yourself to indulge in small amounts, once in a while. Integrating chocolate and other foods you enjoy, in small doses into your daily diet, can help you make your flat belly diet plan successful!

Occasional chocolate treats are not of any great importance, if you are doing everything else right. One or two small pieces of dark chocolate will not ruin your diet. In fact, knowing that you can allow yourself a treat or reward for sticking to a flat belly diet can make those dietary changes a lot easier to live with. And dark chocolate is good for you!

Keep in mind that milk chocolate and white chocolate don't offer the same health benefits as dark (70% or more) chocolate. So if you enjoy an occasional bite of chocolate along with your usual healthy diet, make it dark. Just like the other foods that you put in your body, you want to get high quality chocolate as well. Look for good quality dark, organic chocolate, with few ingredients, in the health food section of your grocery store or at a place like Whole Foods

Maximize Your Flat Belly Journey: Get Powerful Fat Loss Secrets From Key Food And Fitness Experts.
http://velocityhousepresents.com/FlatBellyKitchen

or Trader Joe's. These stores carry a wide selection of dark, delicious, organic chocolate with yummy additions like sea salt, nuts, dried fruits and other scrumptious additions.

Choose dark chocolate with a cocoa content of at least 70% or higher to keep your sugar content low, and the antioxidants high. Any good dark chocolate will list their cocoa content on the package. Generally, chocolates in the range of 70-80% cocoa content have the best taste but have much lower sugar levels than milk chocolate or dark chocolates that are lower than 70% cocoa. Many milk chocolates are only 30% cocoa, and some cheap dark chocolates are only 50% cocoa... and this means that the remaining non-cocoa ingredients are sugar and other junk additives.

Chocolate is made from the beans of the cacao tree, Theobroma Cacao Plant. Cacao is full of flavonoids. These flavonoids are plant-based compounds with powerful antioxidant properties, which means they reduce inflammation, promote healthy arteries, and help fight aging by preventing—and repairing—cellular damage. A small bar of dark chocolate can contain as many flavonoid antioxidants as six apples, four and a half cups of tea, or two glasses of red wine.

Good **dark** chocolate can serve as an appetite suppressant, lower your blood pressure, improve your mood, and add antioxidants. Dark chocolate's bitter taste might help the body regulate appetite, or its higher amount of cocoa butter, with its stearic acid, may make the stomach stay full longer.

Some other great things about chocolate:

• Cacao contains antibacterial agents that can actually fight bacteria in the mouth and tooth decay, but is ineffective if you are eating chocolate with high sugar content.

• Chocolate contains an ingredient that is a mood elevator.

• Cocoa butter in chocolate contains oleic acid, a monounsaturated fat which is good for the heart.

• Chocolate contains magnesium, which helps you feel calm and relaxed, as well as lowering blood pressure.

• Chocolate increases antioxidant levels in the blood.

- Chocolate helps to raise serotonin levels in the brain, resulting in a sense of well-being.

For some people who are sensitive to chocolate, chocolate may have a downside:

1. Chocolate may trigger headaches in those who get migraines.

2. The theobromine in chocolate can cause acne outbreaks. I know, some doctors say chocolate does not cause acne, but it does for me, and probably other people as well.

3. Chocolate is especially toxic to pets, so never share with them.

Go easy on chocolate…save it as a special treat, and just eat a small amount of it at a time.

Personally, I have a sweet tooth, and one of the ways that I've learned to control my sweet tooth over the years is to simply have 1-2 small squares of dark chocolate after a meal.

Because of the rich flavor of dark chocolate, 1-2 small squares is enough to satisfy my sweet tooth while consuming very minimal calories (usually under 50 calories if the squares are small). And all of this while also getting some antioxidant benefits, appetite satisfying benefits from the healthy fats, and MUCH less sugar than most other desserts!

If you want to enjoy the benefits of the powerful antioxidants and fiber in chocolate but don't want the calories, get some organic unsweetened cocoa powder (or raw cacao nibs) and add that to smoothies or other recipes.

Maximize Your Flat Belly Journey: Get Powerful Fat Loss Secrets From Key Food And Fitness Experts.
http://velocityhousepresents.com/FlatBellyKitchen

CHAPTER 23
The Skinny on Tea

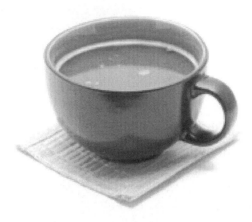

Is green tea or oolong tea good for weight loss?

There has been heavy marketing in recent years for supplements/pills containing either green tea or oolong tea and claiming to be a miracle weight loss aid.

The truth is that there are some minor benefits to green tea, white tea, oolong tea, and black tea in the fat burning process and your metabolism. Just beware of companies that claim tea in a pill to be a "weight loss miracle" or anything where they claim you don't have to change your diet or exercise at all.

However, that doesn't mean there aren't great benefits to these teas, including some benefit in the weight loss department – just realize that teas are best in their naturally brewed form, and you don't need to buy expensive supplements containing tea extracts.

Green tea has received the most attention of all of the Camellia Sinensis plant teas. What is it about green tea? Well, the benefits of green tea are numerous. In fact, if you were to go to PubMed.com and do a search for green tea, you'd find over 2,000 studies performed on green tea and its components. Suddenly everyone is paying attention to green tea! Possible benefits are being investigated for weight loss, cancer prevention, antioxidant activity, cognitive enhancement, general good health and well being, and the list goes on and on.

But what makes green tea an aid for fat loss? First of all, green tea is a source of caffeine, delivered in a more mellow, sustained way than the caffeine jolt of coffee. Caffeine, of course, is a decent fat burner with a well-established track record. Green tea also aids weight loss by increasing the metabolic rate, causing those who use it to experience a small increase in calorie burn (American Journal of Clinical Nutrition). This makes it a decent quality fat burner in and of itself.

However, if that's all green tea did, this would be a pretty short section. Luckily, it provides additional benefits—far beyond what plain caffeine could do. First, it's a powerful anti-oxidant. Yes... just like vitamin C and beta-carotene, and fruits and veggies! But researchers have suggested that the active ingredient (called epigallocatechin gallate, EGCG) may be up to 200 times more powerful than vitamin E as an antioxidant.

Green tea may be useful as a glucose regulator—meaning it slows the rise in blood sugar following a meal. When you keep your blood sugar stable, you cut down on your insulin response, which in turn means more controlled appetite and less stored belly fat! It does this by slowing the action of a particular digestive enzyme called amylase. This enzyme is pivotal in the breakdown of starches (carbs), which can cause blood sugar levels to soar following a meal. This is quite exciting as green tea might be a missing link in proper glucose management.

A recent study also validates green tea's effectiveness. Published in the American Journal of Clinical Nutrition, it indicated the ingestion of a tea rich in catechins leads to both a lowering of body fat AND of cholesterol levels. Double whammy! Additionally, green tea may inhibit fatty acid synthase. Fatty acid synthase is an enzymatic system that is involved in the process of turning carbohydrates into fat. Early animal studies suggest the inhibition of fatty acid synthase can lead to weight loss.

There's also evidence that consuming green tea high in catechins reduces cardiovascular risks in addition to reducing body fat. In short, green tea's weight loss benefits are a result of several mechanisms, including increased metabolism, a positive effect on blood sugar and insulin regulation, and the inhibition of certain enzymes, which are required for the processing of carbohydrates and fats. It also has been shown to lower LDL levels (that's the "bad" cholesterol)

Maximize Your Flat Belly Journey: Get Powerful Fat Loss Secrets From Key Food And Fitness Experts.
http://velocityhousepresents.com/FlatBellyKitchen

as well as triglyceride levels.

Best benefits start with 2-3 cups of tea a day. Not into hot liquids? Make some up and pour it over ice with a little stevia to sweeten it up. There are many types of green tea out there to choose from: some have caffeine, some do not; some are flavored with orange, chai, jasmine, etc. Look for a reputable brand and choose organic when possible.

Remember that white tea, oolong tea, and black tea are all from the same plant as green tea and may have similar benefits, but have simply been studied less than green tea. Each type of tea has unique antioxidants, so there may be additional benefits to mixing up your variety of teas. For example, my favorite healthy drink that I've been making for years is an iced tea mixture where I use some green tea bags, some white tea bags, and some oolong tea bags and make a mixed iced tea, sweetened just ever so lightly with a little stevia. Aside from plain water, this is the healthiest possible drink you can have with your meals or during the day.

In addition, many herbal teas offer a huge variety of antioxidants and are great substitute for sodas, juice, etc. that add empty calories and weight gain. There are berry teas, red teas (aka—rooibos tea), mint teas, chamomile teas, yerba mate, hibiscus teas, etc. All of these teas have additional unique antioxidants not found in other teas and can have benefits. For example, hibiscus teas (which is a herbal form of tea) have been found in studies to help reduce blood pressure. Also, chamomile tea is known for its calming benefits and contains unique phytonutrients that can help to fight the effect of estrogenic pollutants or pesticides inside your body. All of these taste delicious hot or cold, and some are so good and naturally sweet (with 0 calories) they don't need anything else. Try Celestial Seasonings Berry Zinger tea over ice for a delicious refreshing summer drink. One of my favorites!

CHAPTER 24
Create Your Own Flat Belly Kitchen
The Best Veggies and Fruits (buy local whenever you can!)

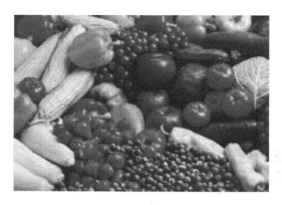

Depending on where you live and what season it is, you may have a bounty of fresh fruits and vegetables grown near you. Check out your local farmer's market, and some grocery stores now even carry local produce.

Always buy local whenever you can. You support your smaller local farmer, and the produce is infinitely fresher than the kind you get that has been shipped for thousands of miles across the country or from other countries. Local produce generally is either organic or close to organic, and has fewer pesticides, herbicides and preservatives on them making them far, far healthier for you.

If you can't find or afford organic, or locally grown, then take a look at this list of foods to avoid for non-organic produce:

Avoid the "Dirty Dozen"
*   Apples
*   Cherries
*   Grapes, imported (Chile) • Nectarines
*   Peaches
*   Pears
*   Raspberries
*   Strawberries
*   Bell peppers
*   Celery

Maximize Your Flat Belly Journey: Get Powerful Fat Loss Secrets From Key Food And Fitness Experts.
http://velocityhousepresents.com/FlatBellyKitchen

- Potatoes
- Spinach and Kale

These foods are the highest pesticide sprayed commercially sold produce. So if you can't get local or organic, try to avoid these in conventional form. They are laden with pesticides, and toxins.

These fruits and veggies are much safer to eat non-organic form:

- Bananas
- Kiwi
- Mangos
- Papaya
- Pineapples
- Asparagus
- Avocado
- Broccoli
- Cauliflower
- Onions

Why does organic cost more? Growing organic food is more labor-intensive. And even though organic food is a growing industry, it doesn't have the economies of scale or government subsidies available to conventional growers. So if you have to buy conventional, you can take some precautions to protect yourself from pesticides:

- Buy fresh vegetables and fruits in season and locally. When long storage and long-distance shipping are not required, fewer pesticides are used.

- Trim tops and avoid the outer leaves and stalks of celery, lettuce, cabbages, and other leafy vegetables that may contain the bulk of pesticide residues.

- Peel and cook when appropriate, even though some nutrients and fiber are lost in the process.

- Eat a wide variety of fruits and vegetables. This would limit exposure to any one particular pesticide residue.

- Purchase only fruits and vegetables that are subject to USDA regulations. Produce imported from other countries is not grown under the same regulations as enforced by the USDA. We import a lot of produce from Mexico and it is best to avoid unless it is organic.

- Wait until just before preparation to wash or immerse your produce in clean water. When appropriate, scrub with a brush. This removes insect residue and dirt, as well as bacteria and some pesticide residues.

- Special soaps or washes are not needed and could be harmful to you, depending on their ingredients. Cool water is perfectly fine.

Other Foods to Stock in Your Kitchen

Ok, now you know the important foods you need to transform your kitchen and your body. There are many other foods, spices and condiments that are also great additions to your flat belly kitchen. Let me give you a partial list of some these items.

Remember, if you don't have junk around the house, you're less likely to eat junk. If all you have is healthy food around the house, you're forced to make smart choices. Basically, it all starts with making smart choices and avoiding temptations when you shop for food.

Once you realize the reasons to avoid the junk and eat the good stuff, you are well on your way to a healthier lifestyle and a lean strong healthy body and a flat belly will be the result, along with oodles of energy and a new outlook on life. Coincidentally, the same foods that help you stay lean are also the foods that are optimal for your health and wellbeing. Amazing!

Let's start with foods to keep on hand in your refrigerator. One or two times a week, load up on fresh veggies. During the summer, visit your local farmers' market frequently and get the freshest, tastiest produce you can get, short of growing it in your own backyard.

If you don't have a farmer's market or farm stand near you, your next best choice is to shop for fresh produce at the grocery store.

Maximize Your Flat Belly Journey: Get Powerful Fat Loss Secrets From Key Food And Fitness Experts.
http://velocityhousepresents.com/FlatBellyKitchen

YOUR SHOPPING LIST

☐ **Vegetables like zucchini, asparagus, onions, fresh mushrooms, spinach, kale, broccoli, Brussels sprouts, red peppers, cilantro, parsley, and more**, to add to omelets, salads, stir-fries, shish kabobs, etc.

☐ **Coconut milk** is another versatile staple to keep on hand. I like to use it to mix in with smoothies, sauces, and broths for a rich, creamy taste. It's also really good in your coffee if you use cream. Not only does coconut milk add a rich, creamy taste to lots of dishes, but it's also full of healthy saturated fat burning fats.

☐ **Cottage cheese, ricotta cheese, plain Greek yogurt and raw cheeses** – Try cottage or ricotta cheese and plain yogurt together with chopped nuts and berries for a great mid-morning or mid-afternoon meal. Greek yogurt is a much better choice than regular yogurt as it has almost twice as much protein as regular yogurt. Raw cheese (grass-fed is the best) is awesome and a rich source of more useable calcium, vitamin K2 for your bones and tons of enzymes.

☐ **Almonds, pecans, walnuts, pistachios, Brazil nuts**—chopped or whole delicious and great sources of healthy fats. Grab a handful for a healthy, filling snack or throw some into your smoothies, salads and veggies.

☐ **Whole eggs** – one of nature's richest sources of nutrients (and remember, they increase your GOOD cholesterol so stop fearing them). Get them free range and organic, if at all possible. Always include the yolks—the richest source of nutrients in the egg.

☐ **Nut butters** – Peanut butter is a bit boring, so get creative and try almond butter, cashew butter, or even macadamia butter for delicious and unbeatable nutrition!

☐ **Salsa** – I try to get creative and try some of the exotic varieties of salsas. Lots of grocery stores now sell this in the fresh produce aisle and it is as delicious and fresh tasting as homemade. Try this on your eggs in the morning for a healthy eye-opener! And remember, the hot peppers in salsa increase your fat burning potential.

☐ **Butter** – Don't believe the naysayers—butter, especially from grass fed cows, adds great flavor to anything and can be part of a healthy diet (just keep the quantity small because it is calorie dense, and NEVER, EVER use margarine, unless you want to assure yourself a heart attack). My favorite grass-fed butter is Kerrygold Irish butter, as all cows in Ireland graze on lush green pastures and are not fed corn.

☐ **Avocados** – Awesome source of healthy fats, fiber, and other nutrients. Try adding them to wraps, salads, on top of omelets, or sandwiches or scooped out of their shell with a touch of fresh lime or lemon juice.

☐ **Whole grain wraps or gluten-free brown rice wraps** (look for wraps and bread with at least 4-5 grams of fiber per 20 grams of total carbs). Remember that it's best to minimize grain intake if fat loss is your goal, so use these sparingly.

☐ **Baby greens, dark green leaf lettuce or red leaf lettuce, romaine, argula, and organic baby spinach** for salads. Make a high protein meal out of your salad by adding some cooked chicken, fish or sliced beef.

☐ **Home-made salad dressing using balsamic vinegar, Udo's Choice Oil Blend, and extra virgin olive oil.** This is much better than store-bought salad dressings which mostly use highly refined soybean oil (highly inflammatory). I often mix up my own concoction of olive oil, balsamic vinegar and fresh lemon juice, chopped fresh basil and thyme, garlic, salt and pepper. Anything you pour this concoction over will really taste terrific!

☐ **Fresh herbs—basil, thyme, oregano, cilantro** – chop on salads, throw into eggs, and garnish meat dishes.

Some of the staples for the freezer:

☐ **Frozen fish – Keep it wild!** Try different kinds of fish each week. There are so many varieties, you never have to get bored. Trader Joe's is a great place to find wild caught frozen fish of all kinds.

☐ **Frozen berries** – during the local growing season, buy fresh, but during the rest of the year, keep a supply of frozen cranberries, blueberries, raspberries, blackberries, strawberries, cherries, etc. to add to cottage cheese, yogurt, or smoothies.

☐ **Frozen veggies** – again, when the growing season is over and you can no longer get local fresh produce, frozen veggies are the best option, since they often have higher nutrient contents even compared to fresh produce that has been shipped across the country. Or buy lots of the fresh veggies when they are in season, and freeze in small portions.

☐ **Frozen chicken breasts or thighs – Organic and free range** if at all possible. Very convenient to cook ahead of time for a quick addition to wraps or sliced on top of a salad for a quick meals. My new favorite is organic, boneless, skinless thighs. The thighs actually have more nutrients and iron since the chicken uses these muscles more. I think they have better flavor and they cost less too.

☐ **Frozen grass-fed meats—bison, beef, lamb, goat, etc.**—Many grocery stores and restaurants are starting to provide these healthier options due to customer demand. If you can't find these meats at your local market, look online. My favorite is U.S. Wellness Meats. And remember, always get 100% grass-fed. If it is 'grain-finished' all the benefits of grass-fed go away.

Now, the staples to keep in the pantry:

☐ **Oat bran and steel cut oats** – higher fiber than those little packs of instant oats that are full of sugar and high glycemic.

☐ **Cans of (full fat) coconut milk** – to be transferred to a container in the fridge after opening.

☐ **A variety of antioxidant rich teas – green, oolong, white, and rooibos** are some of the best.

☐ **Stevia** – the best natural non-caloric sweetener: http://Naturally-Stevia.com

☐ **Organic maple syrup** – none of that high fructose corn syrup Aunt Jemima crap, only real maple syrup can be considered real food. Try a small amount over oatmeal, or added to your post workout shake for muscle-glycogen replenishing carbs.

☐ **Raw honey** – even better than processed honey. It has higher quantities of beneficial nutrients and lots of enzymes. Honey has even been proven in studies to improve glucose metabolism (how you process carbs). I use a teaspoon or so every morning in my tea. Yes, it is pure sugar, but at least it has some nutritional benefits, and a teaspoon of honey is only 5 grams of carbs.

☐ **Brown rice pasta** – Gluten-free and better for you. Brown rice pasta can usually be found in the gluten-free section of the grocery store or health food store and is delicious. Even if you don't have a gluten allergy, it is best to limit your wheat intake. Many people may have problems digesting wheat and gluten and might not even be aware of it. Remember that if fat loss is your goal, we recommend limiting your grain intake overall. So limit even gluten-free items to your once a week cheat meal.

☐ **Quinoa** – An ancient gluten-free, low-glycemic, high protein seed, packed with antioxidants, nutrients and all the essential amino acids. Quinoa has a delicious, nutty taste and is a great substitute for recipes that use rice. Try regular, red or black quinoa.

☐ **Cans of black or pinto beans** – Add to Mexican wraps for the fiber and high nutrition content. Also, beans are surprisingly one of the best sources of youth promoting antioxidants! These are also good thrown into salsas for more protein and fiber.

☐ **Tomato sauces** – Delicious, and as I'm sure you've heard a million times, they are a great source of lycopene. Just watch out for the brands that are loaded with that nasty high fructose corn syrup. Your best and cheapest bet is to stock up on organic tomato sauce and make your own Italian sauce seasoning with salt, pepper, oregano, basil, garlic, and whatever else you feel like throwing in!

☐ **Dark chocolate** (as dark as possible) – This is one of my favorite treats that satisfies my sweet cravings, plus provides loads of antioxidants at the same time. It's still calorie dense, so keep it to just a couple squares, it

Maximize Your Flat Belly Journey: Get Powerful Fat Loss Secrets From Key Food And Fitness Experts.
http://velocityhousepresents.com/FlatBellyKitchen

satisfies without going overboard.

☐ **Organic unsweetened cocoa powder** – I like to mix this into my smoothies for an extra jolt of antioxidants or make my own low-sugar hot cocoa by mixing cocoa powder into hot milk with stevia and a couple melted dark chocolate chunks.

☐ **Sea Salt** – Most grocery stores now carry sea salt and my favorite is the kind you can grind yourself. Nothing tastes better than freshly ground sea salt (there is a huge difference!) on your healthy food, and sea salt is loaded with minerals like magnesium and potassium, and is not nearly as bad for those with reactive high blood pressure. A little goes a long way. New varieties are showing up all time, and they have slightly different flavors. It's all way better than standard iodized salt though so give it a try.

☐ **Variety of Herbal Teas** – Drink hot or cold, sweeten with a touch of honey or stevia if necessary.

CHAPTER 25

Total Transformation Inside and Out!!

So there you have it. Remove the offensive, empty calorie, processed foods and replace them with real, nutrient-dense foods and your body will transform from a fat factory to a fat-burning, flat belly, lean machine. The transformation may not happen overnight, so give it time. But it WILL happen! And in the process, you may find that you no longer want to eat the junk food. Nourishing your body with healthy nutritious REAL food will genuinely satisfy your hunger and give your body what it needs, so no more junk food cravings.

If you generally purchase and eat the foods listed in this book, you will not only begin to change your eating habits for the good, but you will change into a lean strong, energetic, younger-looking you. You will probably also notice some other great benefits to this diet transformation too: smooth, clear skin, shinier, thicker hair, fewer sinus problems, fewer colds and flu, better sex drive, more energy, and quicker recovery time when you work out—to name just a few things. Mentally you should feel sharper, clearer, happier and less irritable too.

I know it isn't realistic to think that you will eat ONLY the foods on this list, but taking smart snacks with you when you are on the run and choosing healthy menu items when dining out should keep you on track. And don't despair if you deviate or have a day when you end up eating poorly. Just get back on track again the next day. My general rule has always been to try to eat healthy 90% of the time and don't beat yourself up for that other 10%!

Just remember this key rule: Eat foods that are minimally processed or not processed at all. Avoid, as much as possible, any food that comes in a package with an ingredient list of more than 3 or 4 items. Eat food that is as close to the way Mother Nature created it as you can. Give your body the fuel it needs and the fat will melt away.

Choose the apple over the packaged applesauce. Eat raw nuts, not the sugar coated, hydrogenated, salty kind from the can. Pick up the raw unpasteurized cheese to nibble on, not the processed stuff in a squirt can. Eat the meat that was raised the way nature intended—grass-fed, free range or wild caught. Eat

Maximize Your Flat Belly Journey: Get Powerful Fat Loss Secrets From Key Food And Fitness Experts.
http://velocityhousepresents.com/FlatBellyKitchen

good fats—the ones that occur naturally in foods, not the processed vegetable oils or trans fats.

Change your shopping habits—buy local at the farmer's markets when you can, shop at healthy grocery stores like Whole Foods (if you have one close to you) or Trader Joe's or the local "mom and pop" health food store. If you have to go to the regular grocery store, try to shop only the perimeter of the store. Most all the other inner aisles of the store are full of shelves lined with processed and packaged foods. No need to be tempted.

Good luck! Enjoy your flat belly, lean body and glowing health! Your friends will all wonder what your secret to success is. And when they ask, have them check out www.truthaboutabs.com for more great articles to totally transform their kitchens and their bodies!

CHAPTER 26

Special Bonus Section by Mike:

The Advanced Nutritional Fat-Burning Blueprint – The 23-day <u>Accelerated</u> Fat Loss Plan

This is the bonus section I promised you. In this section, I'm going to show you all of the nitty gritty details for how I went from 10.2% body fat to 6.9% body fat in only 23 days, while I was preparing for a photo shoot recently.

Now keep in mind that the techniques in this section are NOT for everyone! You really need to be disciplined and these methods are ONLY to be used for 3-4 weeks MAX, and only on occasion, when you really need to accelerate your fat burning to get ready for an event of some sort, maybe a wedding or beach vacation, or whatever it may be.

This is a perfectly healthy method of "peaking" as bodybuilders and fitness models often call it. After all, you can't train with 100% intensity all year, and you can't diet at the strictest levels for 100% of the year either. But working towards a level of "peak condition" is something that is actually a fun goal to work towards once or twice a year.

There is nothing overly "extreme" or "dangerous" about any of these techniques. They are still very healthy eating habits (but just "amped up" a bit), and I didn't use any stimulant-based dangerous fat burner pills at all. All I did during this 23-day fat-burning blast was eat mostly natural whole foods, a few natural supplements, and a few other tricks here and there with spices, teas, etc., along with a strategic training program that was elevated slightly above my normal training levels.

Now keep in mind as we go through some of these choices and methods that some of them may seem like very "minor details" and one of the things I preach all of the time is the big picture. However, in this case, when you combine dozens of these minor details all together at the same time, you can create a powerful fat loss environment in your body, while maintaining lean muscle.

Also, as you read through this, you might think that some of these methods are just going <u>way beyond anal retentive</u>. As a matter of fact, if you tried to do all of these techniques year round, people might think you're mentally insane. But again, this was only a 23-day blast in order to reach a goal VERY quickly. You can do anything you put your mind to that only lasts 23 days. It's actually quite easy.

The reason I was so strict during these 23 days was because of the goal I had set that I was going to do anything it took to reach. I would never do even half of these things on a regular basis as it would make me go crazy. In fact, I've learned how to balance my fitness lifestyle over the years with still having a great social life and being able to go out drinking with friends, eating whatever I want at barbeques or parties on occasion, yet still staying at about 8-10% body fat year round. With this time period though, my goal was to get down to or below 7% body fat, so that's why everything had to be perfect during these 23 days.

I ended up at 6.9% body fat (down from 10.2% body fat) while also maintaining all of my lean muscle during this 23-day cutting cycle! It was fun to actually be working hard towards a specific goal for a few weeks. This alone was quite a motivating factor compared to just "maintaining."

Now let's get into some of the details!

Priorities during this 3-4 week accelerated fat-burning stage:

1. Maintaining your lean muscle to keep your metabolic rate high. Since you'll need to slightly restrict calories, you risk the chance of losing lean muscle during this stage, and that can reduce your metabolic rate, and make fat loss even harder. Top priority is maintaining lean muscle during this stage.

2. Enhance the fat-burning environment in your body to stimulate the release of excess stored body fat.

3. Maximize your metabolism – all of the minor details are going to be aimed at maximizing your metabolism during this time period. We don't have a single day to waste if you have a specific time period goal.

4. Enhance the thermic effect of calorie burning from the food you eat.

5. Reduce stress to minimize negative hormones such as cortisol, and help maximize fat-burning hormones.

6. Maximize the amount of deep sleep that you get, as recovery is going to be super-important during this time period since your training levels will be increased a bit.

The Nitty-Gritty Details

The Type of Weight Training

Since it is so important to maintain lean muscle mass during a "cutting phase" such as this, the weight training needs to be heavy and intense. Light weights and high reps won't cut it when you're in a slight calorie deficit and a slight carbohydrate deficit.

I'm going to mention certain types of exercises in this section, and you should already know how to do most of these exercises, since I'm assuming that you already have a copy of my full Truth about Six Pack Abs program. If there are any exercises you don't know how to do, it's all covered in detail in the full Truth About Abs program, which you can grab a copy at: http://truthaboutabs. com/order.html

Since you'll be slightly reducing overall carbohydrate intake during this period, you don't have the overflowing muscle glycogen at all times to be doing large amounts of single joint isolation exercises. That would simply be a waste of time. Leave the isolation exercises only to a period of time when you're trying to gain weight, and even still only include them as a small portion of the overall workouts.

Sticking to heavy multi-joint exercises is key during the cutting phase—deadlifts, squats, lunges, bench presses, overhead presses, pull-ups, and upper body rows will be the types of main exercises to focus on. One-arm snatches, one-arm swings, and barbell or kettlebell clean and presses can also be great full body additions to the program for their metabolism-boosting effects and stimulation of fat-burning hormones.

I had great results using a 4-day per week weight training program during this cutting phase. Most of the workouts focused on full-body but with different movement patterns each workout to avoid over-training. For most of the weight training exercises, I focused on a fairly heavy weight and moderate rep range, such as 5x5 (5 sets of 5 reps per set, with the 5th rep being very hard to complete on each set)

For example, I did M-W-F-Sat weight workouts during this cycle, and would split it up something like this:

Mon: Bench/Deadlifts supersets; Romanian deadlifts or power cleans; other chest work; finish workout with 10-minute "abs/HIIT circuit" (this circuit will be explained in a minute)

Wed: Squats/pull-ups supersets; lunges or step-ups; other upper back work; 10-min abs/HIIT circuit

Fri: Barbell Clean & Presses supersets with renegade rows; dbell pullovers, dbell squat and presses; 10-minute abs/HIIT circuit

Sat: Shorter workout—kettlebell snatches and swings – both 1-arm and 2-arm versions; kettlebell high pulls

M/W/F workouts were about 1-hr each, and Saturday workouts were short but intense, at about 25 minutes. Because of the time crunch with only having 23 days to prep for this photo shoot, I stepped up the intensity of these workouts by a notch compared to my typical "maintenance" workouts. Also, the 10-minute abs/HIIT circuit that I did at the end of the workout 3 days/week was an add-on that I didn't typically do.

The 10-Minute Abs/HIIT Circuit Explained

I added this 10-minute drill onto the end of my resistance workouts just during this cutting phase.

While we all know that you can't spot reduce abdominal fat by doing ab exercises, there is a reason why I wanted to strategically combine abs exercises into a high intensity interval training circuit…

There have been research findings I've seen lately that indicated slight increases (very slight) in the % of body fat burned from a specific area when the muscles in that area of the body were highly stimulated. The % increases I believe were miniscule and probably don't amount to any significant increased fat loss from a specific area (aka the myth of spot reduction).

The bigger picture as we all know is that exercises that work larger muscle groups of the body like the legs and back burn FAR more overall calories than any ab exercise ever could in the same time period. That's why I've always preached to focus the majority of your workouts on full body drills and no more than about 5 minutes to direct abs training.

However, there is a theory that if you can heavily stimulate the abdominal area with high movement ab exercises such as ab bicycles or floor mountain climbers and then combine those exercises into a circuit with high intensity cardio work, it could possibly slightly increase abdominal fat burning.

While I certainly don't think this is actually "spot reduction" in action, what I do think is that the power of your mind and the placebo effect may actually help you burn fat faster if you strongly think during this entire 10-minute circuit that you are really blasting that abdominal fat. We already know that your mind is very powerful in controlling how your body responds to things as the placebo effect is the ultimate evidence of that power.

So while you're doing these 10-minute abs/HIIT circuits, just keep thinking in your mind how powerfully you're melting away stomach fat... you never know... the power of your mind might actually increase that fat burning. It's not too far-fetched really.

Either way, it was still a killer circuit to end my workouts with!

Here's the way that I structured the 10-minute abs/HIIT circuits:

I would continuously rotate between a floor abs exercise or a stability ball abs exercise and something high intensity such as jumping rope, using a slide board, or doing a 45-60 second "sprint" on a rowing machine. You can really use any apparatus you want, but these were the types of drills that I preferred.

So it would look something like this:

30 seconds abs bicycles
30 seconds super-fast jump rope
30 seconds floor mountain climbers
60 seconds rowing machine
30 seconds abs bicycles
60 seconds on the slide board
30 seconds mountain climbers
30 seconds jump rope
Etc, etc – up to about 10-12 minutes in length for this crazy circuit!

What a way to finish a workout! On the drive home from the gym, I would practice some "ab vacuums." If you don't know how to do "ab vacuums" they are described at this page:

http://www.truthaboutabs.com/flatten-stomach-exercise-trick.html

Manipulating Carbohydrate Intake

No matter how many times you hear all sorts of various "experts" argue low-carb vs high carb, or that "carbs don't matter—it's total calories that matter." Well, I'm going to tell you that carbs DO matter, but my take on it is not extremist in either direction.

Most of the time, I have pretty moderate recommendations for carbohydrates. My stance on the subject could be termed "moderate-low" carbohydrate intake for best fat loss results. I definitely don't agree with the extreme low-carb or no-carb diets that many preach, and I don't agree with a high-carb diet either, as it is VERY hard to lose body fat on a high carbohydrate intake. Even I eat pretty decent amounts of carbohydrates (although I try to reduce grains because of anti-nutrients and gluten in many grains) at most times of the year when I'm just "maintaining".

However, in this section, we're obviously talking about a specific time period where we want accelerated fat-burning, and you can talk to as many bodybuilders, fitness models, and physique competitors as you want (these are people whose JOB it is to get super-lean at certain times), and 99% of them will all tell you that one of the main things they manipulate during a period of cutting body fat is their carb intake.

What I personally did during my 23-day cutting cycle was to eat the MAJOR-ITY of my carbs <u>only</u> on resistance training days, in the morning, and during the post-workout meal.

I was doing resistance training 4 days per week (M/W/F/Sat), so most of my carbohydrate intake was during breakfast on the training days with the work-out being mid to late afternoon... and then the remainder of the carb intake was immediately post-workout. So the day would look something like this:

9am: wake up and breakfast with moderate carbohydrates (maybe 35 g pro-tein, 30 g carbs, 25 g fat)

Noon: small lunch with moderate-low carbohydrates (maybe 25 g protein, 15-20 g carbs, 20 g fat)

3 pm: small snack mostly low GI carbs and healthy fats (such as an apple w/ almond butter)

4:30 pm: High intensity and heavy weight training session for 1-hr

5:45pm: Post workout shake – 2:1 ratio carbs:protein (a couple of my recipes on this page—http://www.truthaboutabs.com/Post-Workout-Nutrition.html) generally about 40 g protein, 75 g carbs, and 5 g fat in this post workout shake.

8 pm: Dinner consisting of a healthy meat such as grass-fed steaks, steamed vegetables with grass-fed cheese, and a large greens salad with avocado (al-most all protein and healthy fats with only fibrous veggies, but no starch-based foods) – no more than about 10 g total carbs with this meal

11 pm: snack such as cottage cheese, cinnamon, stevia, and raw nuts

1 am: get to bed to try to get 8 hours of sleep

There's an important reason I did this. First, in order to be able to do the resis-tance training sessions with enough intensity and heavy enough weights to be able to maintain lean muscle mass during this time period, you need a moderate dose of carbs earlier in the day on a training day. From my experience, if my carb intake is too low on a resistance training day, my workout will suffer and I won't have the energy needed to move heavy weights.

Second, I still wanted to replenish muscle glycogen to help the muscle repair process by consuming a post-workout shake immediately after training. For the remainder of the day with dinner and a late-night snack, it's almost all protein, healthy fats, and fiber that I'm focusing on.

On days that I didn't do resistance training, I focused almost the entire day on mostly protein, healthy fats, and fiber (from vegetables and a fiber supplement, which I'll talk about in a bit). Any exercise I would do on the non-resistance training days would be lighter activities such as hiking or walking, so there wasn't a great need for carbohydrates since explosive exercises and other resistance exercises needing muscle glycogen weren't being done.

Also, being in a slightly carb-deprived state on days when you do light activities such as hiking or walking can help you to increase fat-burning on those days and definitely forces your body to rely mostly on burning fat to provide energy.

So the basic premise during this 23-day cutting cycle was to attempt to keep blood sugar levels under control and prevent high insulin levels MOST of the time, while focusing the majority of my carb intake just on resistance training days in the morning and at post-workout.

One side effect of trying to eat like this (focusing on proteins, healthy fats, and fiber) is that it really forces you to load up on more veggies, and this increases your nutrient density compared to eating breads, pastas, etc and helps to easily control your appetite.

That's one of the most important parts of this whole phase—avoiding grains almost entirely and getting most of your carbs from veggies and some fruits and berries. Grains are more of a weight gaining food as they are just too calorie dense without enough nutrient density (micro-nutrients) for a cutting phase like this. So that's the skinny on manipulating carbs.

Cheat Days?

You might think that since this was only a 23-day cutting cycle, that there's no room at all for any cheat days or even any cheat meals. But you'd be wrong!

Out of the 23 days, I still had 3 cheat days (so about 1 day per week). These weren't full blown cheat days where it was a binge-fest all day long. For the most part, these cheat days were just 1 or 2 extra big meals that were heavy on carbs and fat. The purpose of this was to prevent my body from fighting back and reducing the metabolic rate to preserve calories due to the reduced carbs and reduced calories the other 6 days per week. These cheat meals that were high in carbs and high in fat would stimulate a large insulin spike and help to revamp leptin levels, which will signal to the body that calories are plentiful and increase the metabolic rate.

Again, since this was only 3 cheat days and about 4-5 total cheat meals during this entire 23-day cycle, the cheat meals actually help more than they hurt.

Alcohol Consumption

I don't drink nearly as much as I did in my 20s or in my college days, but even now in my 30s, I still enjoy some drinks out with friends usually about once or twice a week.

However, let's face it, there's nothing about alcohol that is going to help fat loss, and this needed to be a pretty strict 23 days other than the cheat meals I talked about. So I basically tried to avoid all alcohol entirely during these 23 days. I think I drank 2 beers and 2 glasses of wine during this entire 23-day period. This took a little discipline, and there were a couple nights out with friends that I offered to be the designated driver and that made it easier to only drink club soda or unsweetened iced teas while my friends were throwing back a bunch of alcoholic drinks. Overall, it was pretty easy to stay on track in this department.

The Cayenne Trick

Remember that every one of these little details can help slightly, and this was one of those little details. During all 23 days on this cutting phase, I took 2 cayenne pepper capsules during at least 3 meals per day. Cayenne pepper con-

Maximize Your Flat Belly Journey: Get Powerful Fat Loss Secrets From Key Food And Fitness Experts.
http://velocityhousepresents.com/FlatBellyKitchen

tains capsaicin, which helps to create a slight thermogenic effect and increased calorie burn from ingesting the cayenne pepper.

Now keep in mind that we're not talking miracles here, but there is a slight increase in calorie burn from cayenne pepper, and any extra benefit you can get can help when you're doing a cutting phase (even if that extra benefit is the placebo effect in action again!).

Keep in mind that some people have a sensitive stomach, and cayenne pepper (even when taken in capsule form) can give a burning feeling. Personally, it doesn't affect me, so I included it daily in my 23-day plan. You can usually find a bottle of cayenne pepper capsules at any nutrition store for about $5 to $9, so it's cheap.

Cinnamon for Blood Sugar Control

You might have heard about this before… but yes, cinnamon is not only ex-tremely healthy for its antioxidants, but also because it can help control your blood sugar, and maintaining steady blood sugar can keep you burning fat easier.

For this reason, I tried to include cinnamon in any meals that were appropri-ate (such as smoothies, cottage cheese, or in my coffee), and I took about 1-2 grams per day in capsule form if I wasn't including cinnamon in meals. Cin-namon capsules are very cheap ($5 to $7) at most supplement sections, even in grocery stores.

My Protein and Fiber Drink Concoction

When you're doing an accelerated fat burning cycle, protein and fiber are two of the most important things that you need in adequate amounts. Both of them help you to keep hunger under control, and a high protein intake during the cutting cycle can help to prevent catabolism, so you don't lose lean muscle, and you protect your metabolism.

This was another of my secret weapons that I used each day. What I did was use a special protein/fiber drink concoction and have 1 drink each day at a time when I needed to control hunger but didn't want or didn't have time for a full meal. I either used these drinks in the afternoon on non-training days to keep satisfied or I used them at night to keep appetite under control and get an extra dose of fiber and protein.

You can either create your own protein/fiber drink concoction by using your favorite protein powder (not soy protein!) mixed with a good fiber blend (about 3-5 grams of fiber will do the trick). If you don't want to create your own protein/fiber drink, this is the delicious tasting protein/fiber drink that I used, called Fusion. Or go straight to their webpage at: http://natural.getprograde.com/prograde-fusion.html

These protein/fiber drinks were helpful in being a convenient and quick way to ward off hunger and prevent catabolism while keeping calories very low and without any excess carbohydrates.

Chamomile Tea to Aid Fat Loss?

You might be wondering how the heck chamomile tea can aid fat loss, after all chamomile tea has no caffeine, and is actually the exact opposite, in that it is a known relaxant. Well, first of all, you probably have heard about how estrogenic compounds in our environment (from pollution, herbicides, pesticides, petroleum chemicals in household cleaners, etc), and in our food supply (from foods such as soy, beer, and also pesticide residues) can trigger the body to hold onto stubborn belly fat (and can even be one of the causes of "man boobs" in men) if you're exposed to enough of these estrogenic compounds on a regular basis.

These are called xenoestrogens and can make it particularly hard for you to burn off body fat (especially abdominal fat) if you're exposed to these chemicals regularly without protection in your diet. This problem isn't only for men either; these excess estrogenic compounds can create hormone imbalances in women too, and make it even harder to lose stubborn body fat.

This is where chamomile tea can help. Chamomile tea is a potent source of unique phytochemicals and antioxidants that help to fight against any estrogenic compounds that you are exposed to. This can help your body to more effectively burn off stubborn body fat.
Is it a miracle? No, of course not. This is just yet another one of those minor

details, that when combined with all of these other methods, can help you to accelerate fat loss. What I do is simple. I just have a mug of chamomile tea (unsweetened) every night about an hour before bed. It helps to relax me before bedtime anyway, so that's another benefit. At the very least, this is yet another placebo effect that may be helping fat loss, because I believe in my mind that it's working.

Warning: a very small percentage of people can have severe allergic reactions to chamomile, so make sure that you know if you're allergic to chamomile or not if you've never had it before.

Green, White, Oolong Teas & Yerba Mate

As we talked about in earlier chapters in this book, teas such as green, white, and oolong teas all contain varying levels and combinations of unique polyphenols, some caffeine, and other phytonutrients that can slightly increase your fat burning efforts. Plus, yerba mate tea has a unique but very different profile of antioxidants as well. Again, we're not talking miracles, but if you can get a slight advantage, why not take it. Plus, there are many other health benefits from the antioxidant content of teas, so it can't hurt.

What I did during my 23-day blast was make big batches of a gallon at a time of unsweetened iced tea. And then I would drink 3-4 glasses of this tea each day (not too close to bedtime though since it does contain caffeine).

In order to get the maximum benefits and diversity of the polyphenols and other antioxidants, I used a mixture of organic green tea, white tea, oolong tea, and yerba mate tea bags in each batch of iced tea. I would put just a small amount of stevia in these batches of iced tea just for a very lightly sweetened taste. You can get stevia at most grocery stores now or online at: http://Naturally-Stevia.com

Again, even if the fat-burning effect of drinking these teas each day is minimal, any little extra benefit was what I was after. Plus, once again, if my mind believed strongly enough in this, the placebo effect alone may increase the fat burning.

More Organic

While I always recommend consuming as much of your food "organic" as possible, I think this is even more important during a cutting cycle such as this. The reason is that you want to minimize your exposure as much as possible to the estrogenic effects of certain pesticides which can stimulate your body to want to hold onto body fat.

I'd say I probably eat 50-60% of my food normally as organic, but during this 23-day cutting cycle, I was probably at about 80-90% organic.

More Red Meat than Chicken or Fish?

This one may sound unusual, but I actually chose to consume a higher percentage of red meat in the form of grass-fed beef and grass fed bison (and some venison too) during this time period compared to chicken, turkey, or fish.

This may be confusing to you because so many so-called "experts" always tell you that red meat is "bad for you" and to just stick to white meats or fish. Well, there's a specific reason that I chose more red meats (grass-fed) over white meats or fish, and the reason has to do with Conjugated Linoleic Acid (CLA).

CLA is a natural form of healthy fat that occurs in the fat on the meat, and in the dairy from ruminant animals such as cattle, bison, deer, goats, sheep, kangaroo, etc. CLA in natural form has been shown to help aid in burning off abdominal fat and also maintaining or even building lean muscle.

Not many people know this fact, but CLA is actually a natural form of trans fat, but it is FAR different than the artificial trans fats from hydrogenated oils that are so deadly and that you hear all of the negative information about. CLA is actually one of the <u>only healthy trans fats</u> in existence.

<u>Warning</u>: I generally do not recommend CLA supplements as they contain an artificially created form of CLA that is a different CLA isomer compared to the natural CLA isomer that's found in meats and dairy from ruminant animals. The CLA isomer found in CLA supplements is thought by some researchers to possibly have negative effects in the body and is more similar to an artificial trans fat. This is however, controversial and not a lot of studies have been done. The only form of CLA that I personally believe is going to benefit your

Maximize Your Flat Belly Journey: Get Powerful Fat Loss Secrets From Key Food And Fitness Experts.
http://velocityhousepresents.com/FlatBellyKitchen

health and help to reduce body fat is the natural CLA isomers from grass-fed beef, bison, venison, etc or from grass-fed raw milk or cheeses.

Also, grass-fed meats and dairy contain 3-5x the CLA of grain fed meats, so it was grass-fed all the way! And while most cheap whey proteins on the market are made from grain-fed commercial milk that is pasteurized, I've been using a great grass-fed raw whey that also contains significant CLA in it! This is something that most whey proteins don't have. This is where I get it: http://BestGrassFedWhey.com

So that is the reason why I focused more on red meats such as grass-fed beef and bison during this 23-day cutting cycle instead of chicken, turkey, or fish. The extra CLA can really help in accelerating fat burning and preserving lean muscle. I did also eat a good amount of wild salmon during this time for variety, and for the healthy omega 3 fat content, so I didn't solely have red meats as the only meat source.

In fact, one of my "convenience meals" during some of the lunches during this time frame was a mixture of canned wild salmon with a bunch of shredded or diced veggies mixed in (carrots, onions, bell peppers, etc), some spices, and some balsamic vinegar, mustard, and extra virgin olive oil in the mix too. I would just eat this as a form of salmon salad and throw it on top of some greens for a super-healthy and delicious low-carb lunch.

Cruciferous Vegetables

Cruciferous vegetables such as broccoli, cauliflower, kale, Brussels sprouts, cabbage, etc. contain unique and powerful phytochemicals such as indole-3-carbinol (I3C) and other phytochemicals unique to cruciferous veggies that help to inhibit the effect of estrogenic compounds you're exposed to in the environment and your diet. Remember that these estrogenic compounds (xenoestrogens) can increase belly fat or make your body want to hold onto body fat. Therefore, eating cruciferous vegetables each day during this 23-day cutting cycle is likely to help the body fight excess estrogenic compounds and help you to burn body fat faster.

What I did during this 23-day fat blasting cycle was to shift my cooked veggies portion that I usually have with dinner each night and make sure it was a cruciferous vegetable. While I might usually have all sorts of various veggies such as snow peas, string beans, zucchini, peppers, or any number of other vegetables, during this 23-day blast, I focused instead on mostly broccoli, Brussels sprouts, and cauliflower as my main veggie with dinner every night. I would also have a green salad each night too, but the main cooked vegetables I focused on were cruciferous.

This doesn't mean that cruciferous veggies will be my mainstay during every meal the entire year (as I'd probably get sick of them), but for this 23-day blast, my theory was that it could only help and would have a slight advantage over other vegetables.

Onions and Garlic

Onions and garlic also contain potent phytochemicals such as organosulfur compounds that can also help to inhibit the activity of belly fat storing xenoestrogens. Onions and garlic also have many other valuable nutritional benefits, so it's a no-brainer to include them daily in the diet.

Although I usually try to include a fair amount of onions and garlic into my normal diet, during this 23-day blast, I was really conscious of trying to include garlic and onions several times per day in various meals, whether I put them into my eggs in the morning, added to my salmon salad, or as a sautéed side dish to meals. Just another of those minor details that may help accelerate fat burning a slight bit.

Krill Oil

Everyone these days has heard of the benefits of fish oil in helping to increase your omega 3 fatty acid intake, and balance out the excess omega 6 fats. Also, fish oil contains the important EPA and DHA types of omega 3 fats which you can't obtain from plant oils (although there is some small amount of conversion in the body from plant oils).

However, Krill Oil is basically like fish oil on steroids. Krill oil has the benefit of phospholipids which helps your body assimilate and benefit from the omega 3s more effectively compared to standard fish oil.
I used 3 caplets of Krill Oil per day to make sure that I was obtaining enough

phospholipids and omega 3s in the right balance to help aid the body in burning fat efficiently. Also, krill oil has another benefit as it contains a unique and powerful antioxidant called astaxanthan which helps to protect your skin from damage.

Coconut Oil and MCTs

As we've mentioned in other chapters, virgin coconut oil is made up of unique healthy saturated fats called medium chain triglycerides (MCTs), including a specific MCT called lauric acid. Lauric acid has strong benefits on the immune system and is lacking in most modern western diets.

Besides the immunity benefits of lauric acid and the other MCTs in coconut oil, the fats in coconut oil are readily used by the body for energy (easier than most other forms of dietary fat), and can also stimulate your body's metabolism to aid in fat loss. So this is yet another example of a healthy fat that can actually help fat loss.

What I tried to do during this 23-day blast was to use a little bit of coconut oil each day and one of the ways I did this was after I steamed my broccoli or cauliflower, I would then quickly sauté the veggies and a little garlic in about 1 Tbsp of virgin coconut oil. I also always use coconut oil as my oil of choice when cooking eggs. It's the most stable oil under heat and one of the healthiest oils to cook with.

BCAA's and Carnitine

I also used about 3-5 grams per day of branched chain amino acids—BCAAs to help control catabolism, but at very specific times… either in the mornings on an empty stomach before doing morning exercise, or at night before bed. Many studies indicate that BCAAs can be helpful in maintaining lean muscle while restricting calories. And particularly beneficial in preventing catabolism of muscle while doing fasted exercise.

As for carnitine, there appears to be some studies out there that showed some positive benefits to carnitine supplementation to increase fat loss while restricting calories. There are also some conflicting studies that say there is little benefit, if any to carnitine supplementation on fat loss, but these seem to be based on studies with doses that were too small.

However, I got this tip from my good friend and trusted colleague, Jon Benson, and he swears by using liquid l-carnitine during a cutting cycle ONLY, on an empty stomach as it can help aid the body in utilizing fat stores. Jon has a lot of experience in cutting cycles for "peaking," and he was confident that this gives a benefit.

So during my 23-day accelerated fat burning cycle, my strategy was to use about 2 g of liquid l-carnitine first thing in the morning on an empty stomach along with about 2-3 grams of BCAAs and then go for a 30-40 minute brisk walk, bike ride, or hike up the mountain behind my house before eating breakfast.

This goes against my usual philosophy of eating a meal immediately in the morning to reverse the catabolic state that your body is in upon waking in the morning. However, during this 23-day cycle, I wanted to get every possible fat burning advantage as possible, so I made this part of my repertoire about 5 days/week.

Stress Management/Reduction

As you may know, chronic stress is one of the most negative things you can do to your body and your health. And you also may know that stress can chronically elevate cortisol levels, which makes it extremely hard for you to lose body fat.

For that reason, it is essential to find something that helps you to manage and minimize stress in your daily life if you want to maximize your fat burning efforts. This could be as simple as meditating or thinking of a relaxing environment that you love (such as a warm beach) and doing this for a couple minutes every hour, while you're at work, to help manage stress. It also means that you need to program yourself to stay calm in situations that may normally cause you un-necessary stress, such as traffic or rude people.

Or perhaps, a daily bout of yoga, a massage, or something else that helps you reduce stress could be beneficial. For me, I tried to go out on a relaxing hike and get some fresh air on most days when I felt that I had a lot of work to do, and may have been allowing stress to creep in. I live in one of the most beautiful areas of the country (the Colorado Rockies), so it always helps me to relieve stress by getting out and enjoying the scenic beauty and fresh air of the mountains.

Whatever it may be—find that certain activity that you can do that helps you to relieve stress on a daily basis. It can go a long way to helping your health, and your fat burning efforts.

Deep Sleep and Fat Loss

We've all heard a million times that adequate sleep (generally 7-9 hours per night) is essential for just about every aspect of your health. However, during a 23-day cutting cycle like this I was stepping up my training intensity a notch, and also reducing carbohydrates a bit, and overall calories too. Therefore it is even MORE important than ever to make sure to get at least 8 hours of sleep every night to give the body maximum recovery.

Studies show that even partial sleep deprivation, such as 6 hours per night instead of 8 hours per night, can increase cortisol levels, reduce fat-burning and muscle building hormones such as testosterone and growth hormone, and essentially reduce your ability to maximize fat loss and muscle maintenance. There's just no room for error in this type of 23-day cutting cycle if you're serious about your goal, so 8 hours of deep sleep per night is necessary to maximize your results.

The Advanced Strategies—a Little Overboard?

Well, that about does it for all of the nitty gritty details I used to go from 10.2% body fat to 6.9% body fat in only 23 days while prepping for a photo shoot recently. I'll be posting the pictures on my blog in the coming weeks as I don't have them back yet.

Like I mentioned at the beginning of this section, some of this was a little whacky and overly strict, to the point of being anal retentive about every little thing you're doing for several weeks. But again, this was only for 23 days, just in order to meet a specific goal that I had set. I would go crazy if I tried to live my life that way all of the time.

But that's the point of this entire section. You don't have to be this strict all of the time, and you can stay in great shape year-round with a nice balanced fitness lifestyle. But when there are those events like weddings, or beach vacations, or any other event that you want to fine tune your body and cut off some significant body fat in only 3-4 weeks, these advanced strategies can be pretty powerful if you have the motivation and discipline to actually do it!

Maximize Your Flat Belly Journey: Get Powerful Fat Loss Secrets From Key Food And Fitness Experts.
http://velocityhousepresents.com/FlatBellyKitchen

CHAPTER 27
Buying Guide

- **Grass-fed beef, bison, veal, lamb, goat, free range chicken, grass-fed raw cheeses, grass-fed butter and more:** The best source of high quality grass-fed meat, grass-fed raw cheese, grass-fed butter, free range chicken, humanely raised pork, wild caught fish, nutraceuticals, organic nuts, snacks, and more is U.S. Wellness Meats at http://healthygrassfed.2ya.com

  This company ships across the country and in most places, you will receive your order at your door in 2-3 days. Your meat comes vacuum packed and frozen in insulated cold cartons, unless ordered fresh. This may be some of the best tasting meat you have ever had! This company cannot be beat for high quality, grass-fed meats, cheese and snacks. U.S. Wellness Meats also carries a great low sugar, high fructose corn syrup free sports water that fuels active lifestyles.

- **Wild Caught Fish:** Best online source for a great variety of delicious, wild caught sustainable salmon and high omega 3, certified pure, sushi-grade fresh and frozen fish is Vital Choice Seafood. Check out the tabs "Doctors Top Choices" and "Product Starter Packs" for great ideas on what to order. Also try Alaskan Sablefish for a rich, delicious melt-in-your-mouth super healthy, high omega 3 treat. Trader Joe's is also a great place to buy small packages of wild caught frozen fish of various kinds, as well as your local grocery store. Look for "wild caught" not "farm-raised."

- **Nuts**: Obviously the grocery does carry nuts, but try to find the raw nuts, or those without added omega 6 oils, which kind of defeat the purpose of eating them. One of the best places to find great selections of nuts, trail mix, etc. at great prices is Trader Joe's.

- **Raw Milk:** go to http://www.realmilk.com/where1.html Find your state and click on it to search for dairy farms near you. Some farms will ship to your home or deliver close to where you live. Some of these farms also carry free range organic eggs, grass-fed meats, and other items as well.

- **Stevia**: is now readily available at most grocery stores. The more pure version of Stevia is usually sold in health-food sections of grocery stores or healthier food stores like Trader Joe's and Whole Foods. Lots of times Stevia is placed in the 'supplement' aisle, because of FDA rulings. Expect to see Stevia or derivatives of Stevia in mainstream soft drinks, frozen treats, and other low calorie sweetened items. That still doesn't mean these are great items to be ingesting, but possibly less bad than before!

- **Gluten-free brown rice pasta and gluten-free brown rice wraps:** Grocery stores are really starting to pick up on the gluten-free trend, and many actually may have a gluten-free section in the store. Otherwise check your regular pasta aisle for brown rice or whole wheat pasta. Trader Joe's and Whole Foods have a big variety of gluten-free brown rice pastas of all different shapes and sizes. Just remember that if fat loss is your goal, grains should be kept to a minimum.

- **Miscellaneous:** Most grocery stores now carry the rock sea salt in the little grinder. Rather than buy a new grinder with salt in it every time, you can buy a bigger container of sea salt in the larger crystal size and just fill up the grinder. This saves money and keeps you stocked with great tasting salt.

- Healthier food stores carry great **dark chocolate**, but many grocery stores now carry decent dark chocolate as well. Remember that milk chocolate is more fattening, contains more sugar, and not as good for you, so stick with dark chocolate that is at least 70% cocoa, with no additives or preservatives.

- **Coconut oil**: Whole Foods or your health food store. Your grocery store may also have it in the health foods aisle. Be sure it is in its natural state, and not refined or hydrogenated.

- **Healthy energy bars:** Whole Foods, Trader Joes, your local grocery store's health food aisle, or order some amazing raw food bars here—Dale's Raw Food bars -these are some delicious raw protein bars with loads of fiber, and great taste too! Another bar that is more of a "snack bar" and is very tasty, but not necessarily high in protein are these: http://natural.getprograde.com/cravers

Special Bonus
Flat-Belly Recipes

Huevos Rancheros

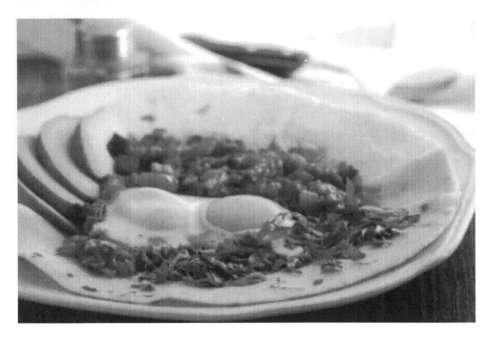

The avocado is full of healthy monounsaturated fats, which actually help to keep blood sugar stable, and to turn on the body's fat-burning ability for the day. You are more satisfied—and you burn fat better all day with the addition of avocado to your breakfast.

<u>Ingredients</u>

- 1 Tbsp of grass-fed butter
- 1 small can mild green chili peppers, chopped
- 1 14 oz can black beans, drained
- ½ cup grated raw grass-fed cheese (optional)
- 1 small chopped tomato or fresh salsa (you can purchase fresh salsa at grocery store)
- Juice of one lime
- Handful of cilantro leaves, chopped

- Sliced avocado
- 4 eggs
- Sea salt and fresh black pepper
- 4 brown rice or sprouted wheat tortillas (optional)

Directions
Melt butter in skillet over medium heat and fry eggs sunny-side up or over-easy in grass-fed butter. In another small pan, add beans and green chilies and heat up until warm.

Layer tortilla, beans, and eggs; top with a sprinkle of grated cheese if desired, and a big spoonful of salsa, a few slices of avocado and a generous amount of chopped cilantro. Serves 2-4.

Dutch Baby (neither Dutch, nor a baby—but certainly delicious!)

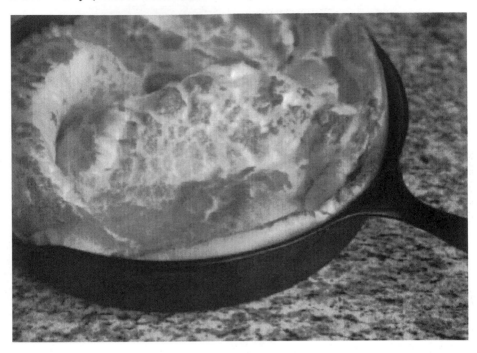

I am not a big advocate of using grain-based flours of any type, but occasionally I allow exceptions *if* I am planning on a hard workout, because food for high-energy endurance requires a mix of good fats, protein and low-glycemic carbs.

I will also make an exception if the flour is gluten-free, whole grain flour. I use organic brown rice flour in this recipe so the finished product is not quite as fluffy and impressive looking as if you used regular processed white flour, but it is way healthier and every bit as good!

Coconut flour works too, but generally it works better if you blend it at least 50-50 with brown rice flour. Coconut flour tends to soak up liquids due to its high fiber content, so be sure to add a ¼ cup or so more milk. And while it will taste every bit as good, coconut flour is a bit heavier and the pancake will not rise as much or be as pretty as with rice flour.

This recipe can be adapted for various sizes and servings. If you would like a smaller version, just cut the recipe in half and use 2 or 3 eggs, ½ cup each of flour and milk and 3 Tbsp of butter. You can use a smaller pan, or just have a thinner, crispier version in the same large pan. Top with fresh berries like strawberries, blueberries, or blackberries.

Ingredients

- 4 eggs
- ½ to 1 cup brown rice flour or a mixture of coconut and brown rice flour
- ½ to 1 cup of raw whole milk, hemp milk, coconut milk or almond milk
- ¼-1/3 cup of grass-fed butter
- Pinch of sea salt
- 1 wedge of lemon

Directions

Heat oven to 425 degrees F. Place butter in 10-12" oven safe skillet or frying pan. Place pan in hot oven to melt butter, 5-7 minutes (I use an iron skillet for this). While the butter is melting in pan in the oven, mix up the batter.

In a blender, add eggs and blend for about 1 minute. Slowly add in some of the flour and some of the milk, blending as you go. If you like, you may add a small bit of vanilla, and a pinch of salt. Blend for another minute or two on high, then remove the HOT pan from the oven and pour in the batter.

Bake in oven for 16-20 minutes, until golden-brown. The Dutch Baby will be fluffy and coming up the sides of the pan or bubbly in the center. Remove from the oven, squeeze fresh lemon over it, sprinkle with cinnamon and serve with fresh fruit like blueberries, strawberries, etc. If fresh fruit is not in season, frozen pureed berries are just as good and full of all the antioxidants and nutrition of fresh fruit. Serves 4-6.

Maximize Your Flat Belly Journey: Get Powerful Fat Loss Secrets From Key Food And Fitness Experts.
http://velocityhousepresents.com/FlatBellyKitchen

Spinach-Egg Mini Quiche Cups

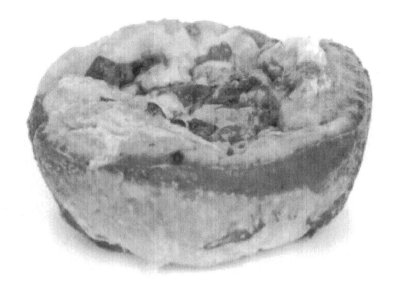

This is a great meal to make ahead and keep on hand in the fridge for a fast, healthy, high protein, low glycemic, fat-burning meal or snack. Be sure and use all the egg yolks as well as the whites, because the yolks contain most of the healthy fats, vitamins, minerals and nutrients.

You can add virtually any type of vegetable to this, just cut them up in smaller pieces. Any way you go, you will be adding powerful antioxidants and vitamins and minerals. Try spinach or kale, chopped mushrooms, sweet red peppers, asparagus, or zucchini.

Ingredients

- 6 large eggs, beaten
- 1 small package of frozen organic spinach
- ½ cup of chopped red pepper, asparagus, or other vegetable
- ½ cup or so of shredded raw, grass-fed cheese (optional)

150

- ¼ cup of minced onion
- Dash of Tabasco, or other hot sauce, or red pepper flakes
- Sea salt
- 1-2 slices of natural, nitrite/nitrate-free ham, sausage or bacon if desired, diced
- Muffin pan sprayed with nonstick cooking oil for 12 servings

Directions

Heat oven to 350 degrees F. Spray muffin pan with cooking spray. Thaw and drain the spinach. You can wring out the spinach with your hands and get most of the excess liquid out of it.

Mix all ingredients in with the beaten eggs, and pour into muffin cups. Bake in 350 degree oven for 20 minutes, or when a knife inserted comes out clean. Cool and serve.

Can be refrigerated and re-warmed in a pan (low heat with lid on) to reheat. Great topped with fresh salsa and avocados! Makes 12.

White Chicken Chili

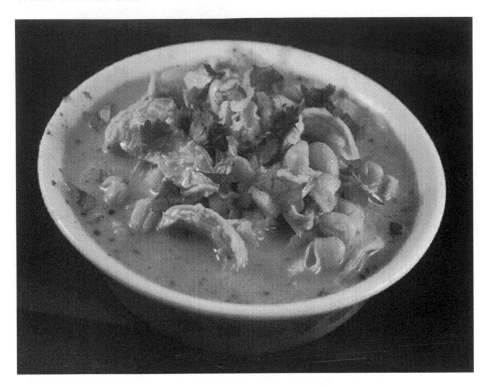

A delicious variation of regular chili that is lighter and uses chicken instead of beef. This recipe tastes especially good with generous amounts of cumin and when you see the health benefits of cumin, you will enjoy its taste even more!

Cumin seeds stimulate the secretion of pancreatic enzymes, which are necessary for optimal digestion of proteins, fats, and carbohydrates, and help the body use the nutrients in the food you eat. Cumin seeds also have anti-cancer properties as well. In one study, cumin was shown to protect against stomach or liver tumors.

Cumin, like cinnamon, helps keep blood sugar levels stable, which means cumin is great for diabetics or pre-diabetics, and it means less chance of weight gain and excess body fat. Cumin has been proven to work as well as some commonly used diabetic drugs at regulating insulin and glycogen. Cumin is also a very good source of iron, vitamin C and vitamin A, which benefit

the immune system.
Add cumin liberally to this recipe!

Ingredients

- 2 lbs. organic chicken breasts, or boneless skinless thigh meat
- 1-2 Tbsp extra virgin olive oil
- 2 cloves of garlic, minced
- 2 cans white beans
- 2 medium onions, diced
- 1 small can mild green chili peppers, chopped
- 1 cup chopped fresh cilantro
- 2 cups chicken stock or more or less to taste
- 2-4 tsp cumin powder
- 1 tsp chili powder
- Sea salt and pepper
- Red pepper flakes, if desired

Directions

Cook chicken in large soup pan in extra virgin olive oil with garlic and onions. Remove the chicken from the pan and allow it to cool.

When cool, shred with a fork. Add all ingredients to a large pan and simmer over medium-low heat. Cook for about 30 minutes or more, stirring occasionally.

Garnish with a dollop of avocado slices, organic sour cream, organic grass-fed cheese, and a generous handful of cilantro—or all of the above. Serves 4 or more.

The Best Black Bean Soup Recipe, Ever

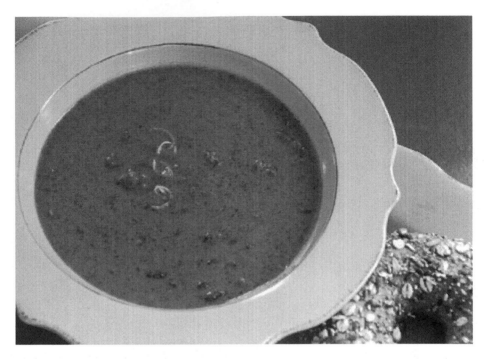

Okay, so you've heard black beans are good for you? I bet you don't know how nutritionally powerful these little guys can be! The dark color of the beans comes from a potent group of antioxidants called anthocyanins, the same fantastic flavonoids found in nutritional rock stars like blueberries, cranberries, red cabbage, and red beets.

Black beans actually have the highest levels of antioxidants of beans, and as much as the antioxidant-loaded cranberry. A cup of black beans provides half your daily requirement for fiber, helping reduce hunger cravings. They're especially rich in soluble fiber—the kind that helps to lower LDL cholesterol and stabilize blood sugar levels.

Black beans are one of the best sources around for the trace mineral molybdenum. You may not realize it, but this vital mineral is necessary for the metabolism of fats and carbohydrates, protein synthesis, helps our bodies use iron, protects against cancer, prevents anemia, promotes a feeling of general well-being, helps to prevent sexual impotence in men, and helps to prevent tooth

154

decay. Whew! That's a lot of good stuff!

Black beans are also a good source of protein, folate (vitamin B6) and magnesium to maintain energy levels.

Ingredients
- 1 ½ cups of black beans rinsed and soaked 6-8 hours or overnight OR
- 2 cans of organic black beans, drained and rinsed
- 1 small onion, diced
- 2 garlic cloves, minced
- Sea salt
- Sprinkle of hot pepper flakes
- 2 tsp of cumin
- 2 cups of water or chicken stock
- Fresh salsa (I find this in the produce aisle of my grocery store), or you can use the kind that comes in a jar if you can't find the fresh stuff.
- Garnish with fresh cilantro, sliced avocado, and bacon!!

Directions
If using dried beans, rinse beans and soak overnight. Drain the water they are soaked in, and add fresh water, and bring to a boil. Skim off any foam that appears on top. Simmer beans for about an hour or until tender and drain beans. Sauté onions and garlic in extra virgin olive oil in separate pan, then add cooked beans. If using canned beans, add them at this point.

Add other ingredients, and cook an additional 20-30 minutes or more. This soup can be blended in a blender for a creamy, thick texture if desired. Cool soup and blend about half, then add to the rest of the soup. Serve with a dollop of sour cream, avocado slices and cilantro. Serves 4.

Hearty Vegetable Beef Soup

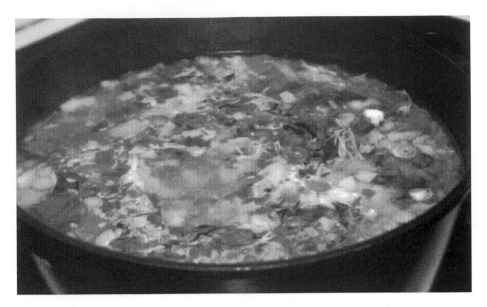

This is one of those soups you can make in a variety of ways, using whatever fresh ingredients are available and in season at the time.

I try to always use grass-fed beef, as it is far superior in nutrients and healthy fat content to commercially raised grain-fed beef, plus it tastes way better than conventional meat!

Be sure and add in a handful of blended kale, Swiss chard, or other hearty greens to supercharge this delightful, nutritious soup even more.

Ingredients
- 2 Tbsp extra virgin olive oil
- 1 lb grass-fed beef stew meat, or boneless chuck, brisket, tri-tip steak, sirloin steak, etc., cut into small chunks
- 1 large yellow or red onion, chopped
- 2-3 garlic cloves, minced
- 2 carrots, chopped
- 2 organic celery stalks* chopped
- 2 red-skinned potatoes, scrubbed but unpeeled, cut into chunks
- 1 large can (28 ounces) crushed plum tomatoes, with juices

- ½ lb green beans, trimmed
- 1 small summer (or yellow) squash, quartered and chopped
- 1 small zucchini, quartered and chopped
- 2 tsp oregano
- 2 Tbs. chopped fresh flat-leaf parsley
- Salt and freshly ground pepper, to taste
- Red pepper flakes, optional

Directions

In a large saucepan over medium heat, add extra virgin olive oil and beef. Cook beef until slightly browned. Add the salt and pepper, oregano, garlic, onion, carrots and celery; cover the pan and cook, stirring occasionally, until the onion is softened, about 5 minutes.

Add 4 cups of water, potatoes, tomatoes, green beans, squash, zucchini, and greens and simmer, partially covered, for 1 hour. Stir in the parsley and season with salt and pepper. Serves 4 to 6.

Note: I sometimes like to spice this soup up a bit and add a touch of chili powder, cayenne and cilantro for a Southwestern twist.

Conventionally grown celery is highly sprayed with dangerous pesticides. Always buy organic celery if at all possible.

Garden Fresh Gazpacho

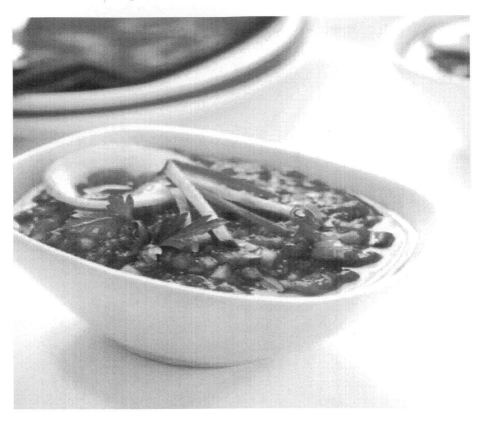

Gazpacho is the perfect soup for summer. Refreshingly cold on hot summer days, this classic Spanish cold tomato soup combines the best of summer's most nutrient and antioxidant-rich vegetables.

This soup is always best when fresh vegetables are at their peak and locally picked, if possible. The best ingredients usually come from local farmer's market with vine ripe tomatoes bursting with real tomato flavor, and fresh home-grown vegetables. Tomatoes are one of those vegetables of summer, when freshly picked and vine-ripened, that have no comparison to those pallid, taste-less globes in the supermarket.

Lycopene is one of the outstanding ingredients in tomatoes that make them so very good for you. Lycopene is effective at preventing cancer including colorectal, prostate, breast, endometrial, lung, and pancreatic cancers. And organic tomatoes deliver three times the lycopene as conventionally grown tomatoes.

When lycopene is eaten with other foods that contain fats, such as avocado, or extra virgin olive oil, it is absorbed even better!

Tomatoes are also excellent source of vitamin C and vitamin A. These antioxidants travel through the body neutralizing dangerous free radicals that could otherwise damage cells and cell membranes, causing inflammation that contributes to heart disease, diabetic complications, asthma, and colon cancer. And all the other fresh veggies in this soup are packed with super powered antioxidants, vitamins and minerals as well! Gazpacho is like eating a liquid salad!

This recipe does not need exact ingredients, so if you have a handful of fresh kale or a garden fresh zucchini, by all means, throw it in!

Ingredients

- 4-6 ripe organic, red tomatoes of any variety, quartered
- 1 red onion, quartered
- 1 cucumber, peeled, seeded, chopped in large pieces
- 2-3 stalks celery, chopped
- 2 carrots
- 1 sweet red bell pepper (or green) seeded and halved
- 1-2 cloves garlic, chopped
- 1-2 Tbsp fresh parsley
- 1 tsp or more of cumin
- Pinch of red pepper flakes, to taste
- 1/4 cup extra virgin olive oil
- 2-3 Tbsp freshly squeezed lemon juice
- 1 tsp raw sugar or honey
- Sea salt and fresh ground pepper to taste
- 1 tsp Worcestershire sauce
- 2-4 cups V-8 or tomato juice
- Cilantro, chopped for garnish
- Avocado sliced, for garnish

Maximize Your Flat Belly Journey: Get Powerful Fat Loss Secrets From Key Food And Fitness Experts.
http://velocityhousepresents.com/FlatBellyKitchen

Directions

Combine all ingredients. Blend at low speed, leaving the soup somewhat chunky. This can be made ahead of time and placed in a glass storage container with a lid and refrigerated overnight, so the flavors blend better. Garnish with sliced avocado, a handful of cilantro or whatever suits your fancy. To add some protein, throw in some cooked shrimp or anchovies (rich in omega 3 fats). Serves 4.

Native American Toasted Pecan Soup

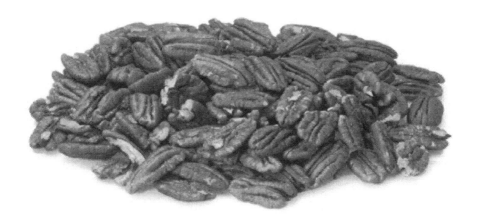

Pecan soups were actually a staple of the Native Americans. Pecans contain more than 19 vitamins and minerals, including vitamin A, B vitamins, vitamin E, calcium, potassium, magnesium, zinc and oleic acid (the same healthy fat that is in extra virgin olive oil). Pecans are also a natural, high-quality source of protein with few carbohydrates, and no cholesterol.

The antioxidants help protect against cell damage, cancer and heart disease. Eating a handful of pecans every day can help protect the nervous system, and may delay the progression of age-related neuron degeneration, which is part of diseases like Alzheimer's, Parkinson's, and amyotropic lateral scle- rosis (ALS). The naturally occurring antioxidants in pecans also contribute to heart health and disease prevention. Pecans contain different forms of the antioxi-dant vitamin E, many of them with antioxidant abilities.

Studies show that eating pecans decreases LDL (bad) cholesterol in the blood by as much as 33 percent. And studies show that nut consumption increases the body's fat-burning metabolism and helps you feel full.

Spicing this soup up with chili powder and cayenne will actually speed up your metabolism—making you more energetic and helping you burn fat even

better. This rich, creamy version is satisfying, packed with nutrients and full of flavor.

Ingredients
- 2 ½ cups of pecans
- 2 Tbsp of extra virgin olive oil
- 1 large onion, chopped
- ¼ cup real maple syrup
- 1 Tbsp chili powder
- 2 cloves garlic, minced
- 3 cups free-range chicken broth or vegetable broth
- 4 sprigs fresh thyme
- 1 cup raw, unpasteurized whole milk, or coconut milk (full fat version in can)
- ¼ cup chopped green onions for garnish

Directions
Preheat oven to 350 degrees F. Spread pecans on baking sheet and toast 7 to 10 minutes or until browned and fragrant. Cool a few minutes and coarsely chop.

Heat extra virgin olive oil in large saucepan over medium heat and add onion and sauté about 5 minutes. Add 2 cups of pecans, maple syrup, chili powder, and garlic. Cook 2-3 minutes. Add broth, thyme, and bay leaf, 4 cups of water and sea salt and pepper to taste.

Cover and simmer 2 hours. Remove thyme sprigs and bay leaf and puree soup in batches in blender. Return to pot and stir in milk or coconut milk and reheat. Garnish with cheese and green onions. Serves 4.

World's Healthiest Cheese Steak Sandwich from Mike

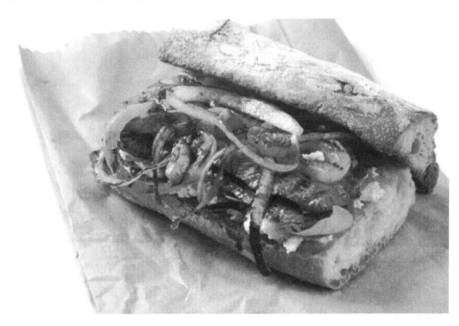

Between the powerful antioxidants in the onions and mushrooms, the medium chain triglycerides (a fat-burning, energy producing type of fat) in the coconut oil, the fat-burning CLA in the grass-fed cheese and grass-fed beef, and the diversity of nutrients in the sprouted grain roll, you could call this a "body-sculpting cheese-steak" sandwich.

If you are going to use a roll, I recommend Ezekiel sprouted grain rolls, which are a mix of about 10 different sprouted grains with no refined flour. As you may know, I'm not a huge fan of eating grains, but if you're going to do it, sprouted grain bread (or rolls) is one of the best options.

If you can't find the Ezekiel brand, most health food stores have other types of sprouted grain bread, but if you can't find sprouted grain bread, try to find a whole grain bread with the highest fiber content as a next best option. Gluten-free is also a great option as well. And for those on a Paleo diet, these are great without a bun—just use your fork instead!

Use a good quality grass-fed beef. As you may already know, grass-fed meat contains more of the healthy fats like omega 3 fatty acids, and CLA (conjugated linoleic acid).

The cheese is raw cheese from grass-fed dairy cows. Grass-fed dairy is also a great source of beneficial fat burning CLA and vitamin K2.

Ingredients
- Ezekiel sprouted grain rolls
- 1 lb or so grass-fed sirloin, ribeye, tri-tip, or skirt steak, sliced thin while still slightly frozen
- 2-3 slices of raw Colby, Monterey Jack or Gouda cheese from grass-fed cows
- Organic Vidalia onions and baby portabella mushrooms

Directions
Sauté the Vidalia onions and mushrooms in a bit of grass-fed butter along with the thin slices of steak until tender and steak is done.

Use a raw longhorn, Colby, or Gouda cheese from grass-fed cows as well. Grass-fed dairy is also a great source of beneficial fat-burning CLA, as well as being easier to digest—especially for those with dairy allergies.

Pile on bun and top with slices of cheese and voila... you now have the **healthiest cheese steak sandwich on the freakin' planet!** But more importantly, it is darn delicious too! Serves 2-4.

Spectacular Beef Fajitas

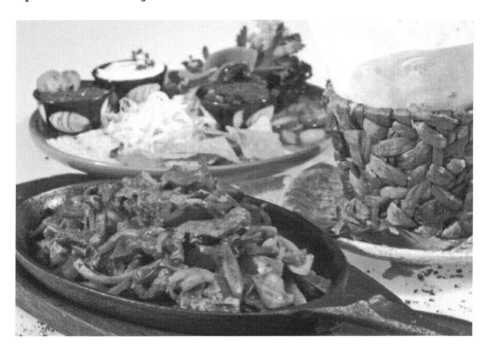

I use a grass-fed inside skirt steak cut for this recipe. It is thin and easy to slice up before marinating and tender and delicious when cooked. The grass-fed meat contains far more healthy fats than conventional beef, including cancer-fighting and fat-burning Conjugated Linoleic Acid (CLA) and omega 3's. In addition, grass-fed or organic meat does not contain all the pesticide residue, antibiotics and hormones that conventional meat contains.

The bell peppers contain plenty of vitamin C and antioxidants; the onions and garlic are loaded with cancer-fighting enzymes, and immune-enhancing, anti-inflammatory power of quercetin, which not only helps you fight off colds and flu, but allergies as well. Tomatoes contain protective lycopene, carotenoids, vitamin A, vitamin C and potassium, which protect against free radical damage, and cancers.

When you add the guacamole, you add even more super-nutrients. Avocados contain an amazing variety of phytonutrients, including key healthy fat-burning fats like alpha-linolenic acid (an essential fatty acid) and oleic acid. Avo-

Maximize Your Flat Belly Journey: Get Powerful Fat Loss Secrets From Key Food And Fitness Experts.
http://velocityhousepresents.com/FlatBellyKitchen

cados are also a good source of vitamin K and copper as well as fiber, vitamin B6, vitamin C, folate, copper and potassium. And to top it all off, the extra spices in this recipe exponentially multiply all the antioxidants and nutrients in everything!

Meat
- 1 lb or more grass-fed skirt steak, sliced into thin (1/4") slices
- 1 large sweet red onion, sliced
- 1 red bell pepper and 1 yellow bell pepper, cut in slices

Marinade
- Juice of 1 medium lime or 1 ½ small limes
- ¼ cup extra virgin olive oil
- ¼ cup Worcestershire sauce
- ¼ soy sauce
- 2-4 garlic cloves, minced
- 2 tsp cumin powder
- 1 Tbsp of Frank's Red Hot sauce or a few sprinkles of hot pepper flakes or cayenne

Guacamole *(Measurements are approximate, adjust to taste)*
- 1-2 whole ripe avocados (should just yield lightly to touch, but not too soft)
- 2-3 Tbsp of minced red onion
- 2 cloves of garlic, minced
- 1 small tomato, chopped
- Juice of one fresh lemon or lime
- Handful of fresh cilantro, chopped
- Sea salt, to taste
- Optional—1 small jalapeño, minced, with seeds and inside ribs removed (use gloves or wash hands if you handle it) or some red pepper flakes
- Brown rice or regular soft tortillas, heated till just soft and warm. (Optional)
- Generous amounts of chopped fresh cilantro for garnish
- Red leaf or romaine lettuce, chopped in thin slices

Directions
Mix up marinade in a shallow glass container, add in slices of beef, pepper

and onions. Cover and marinate 2-4 hours or overnight in refrigerator. Drain off half the marinade and discard, and cook remaining marinade, meat and vegetables in skillet over medium heat until meat is done and vegetables are tender, and liquid is mostly gone. Squeeze fresh lime or lemon over the meat and veggies when done, and garnish with a fist full of chopped cilantro.

Serve with black beans, salsa, lettuce, guacamole and brown rice (gluten-free) tortillas—which are optional, in my opinion. Serves 4.

Maximize Your Flat Belly Journey: Get Powerful Fat Loss Secrets From Key Food And Fitness Experts.
http://velocityhousepresents.com/FlatBellyKitchen

Healthy Hearty Beef Burgundy

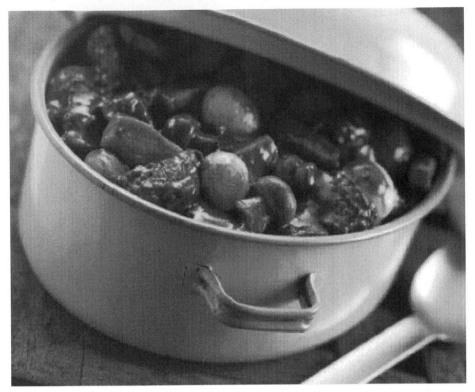

A hearty, filling meal with tender, juicy, grass-fed meat and mushrooms.

This French dish is essentially a beef stew. But the slow cooking in the oven creates something even more magical than just beef stew. The rich aroma fills the kitchen with a tantalizing fragrance, and the broth intensifies and thickens into a velvety sauce. The beef becomes tender beyond belief, and the stew is rich, satisfying and comforting. It's the perfect meal.

The recipe is not complicated, but from start to finish takes close to four hours, because of the cooking time. This dish keeps well, so consider making it over the weekend for dinner, and saving the leftovers for lunch during the week.

Mushrooms add a great earthy, rich flavor, and plenty of nutrients. Mushrooms are a huge source of potassium and contain as much or more than a banana or glass of orange juice.

A serving of mushrooms is an excellent source of copper, which is an important mineral for metabolism. Mushrooms contain rich amounts of riboflavin, niacin, and selenium. Selenium is very valuable in protecting the body against many cancers, as well as helping the thyroid gland (which has a lot to do with your metabolism and energy) function properly.

Mushrooms, especially fresh white button mushrooms, possess chemicals that inhibit an enzyme involved in excess estrogen production in men and women (which results in weight gain), and also have an enzyme that converts testosterone to DHT—which is important for strength and lean muscle mass, as well as increasing your fat burning ability.

Carrots, onions and garlic add antioxidants to power up your immune system, and thyme is excellent for coughs, colds, chest congestion, bronchitis and asthma.

Ingredients

- 2-3 lbs of grass-fed beef stew meat, sirloin, or chuck roast, cut into 1" cubes
- 1/4 lb nitrite-free bacon
- 4 Tbsp grass-fed butter
- 1 ½ tsp salt
- ¼ tsp pepper
- 2 Tbsp brown rice, coconut or almond flour
- 2 carrots, sliced
- 1 onion, sliced
- 1 Tbsp tomato paste
- 2 cloves garlic, finely chopped
- 1 Tbsp fresh thyme (or 1 teaspoon dried)
- 1 Tbsp fresh parsley, finely chopped
- 1 bay leaf
- 3 cups full-bodied red wine
- 2 ½ cups beef stock
- 1 lb white button, crimini, or shiitake mushrooms
- 2 cups cooked quinoa
- ½ cup of fresh parsley, chopped

Directions

Preheat oven to 325 degrees F.

Cut the bacon into short strips. In a deep saucepan, sauté the bacon with 1 Tbsp of butter until bacon is cooked but not crispy. Sprinkle beef with salt, pepper and flour and add to pan with bacon. Brown meat. Set bacon and meat aside in a casserole baking dish.

In the saucepan on the stove, add 1 Tbsp butter to the pan that bacon and meat were cooked in, and sauté the carrots and onion until tender, about 8 minutes.

Add tomato paste, mushrooms, garlic, thyme, parsley, bay leaf. Stir in the wine and beef broth and bring to a gentle boil, simmer for 3-5 minutes, and then pour over the meat in the casserole pan.

Cover, and bake in oven for about 2 and 1/2 hours. The liquid should be gently bubbling the whole time. You'll know it's done when the meat is so tender that it easily pulls apart with a fork. Garnish with parsley and serve over quinoa or brown rice. Serves 4.

Indian-Style Beef Kabobs with Cilantro Sauce

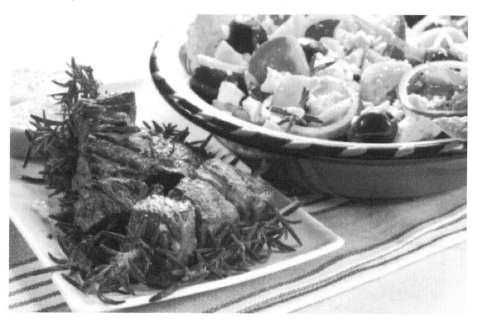

Ingredients

- 1 bunch of fresh cilantro (2 cups cilantro leaves)
- 1 small onion peeled
- 2 cloves garlic, peeled
- 1 small green chili pepper trimmed and halved
- 1 2 inch piece of fresh ginger, peeled
- 1 1/4 tsp sea salt
- 4 Tbsp olive oil
- 3 Tbsp fresh lime juice (juice of one lime)
- 1/2 curry powder
- 1 1/2 lb rib-eye steak, cut into 24 one inch chunks
- 1 medium onion, peeled
- Naan bread or pita bread or flour tortillas

Directions

Place the cilantro, onion, garlic, chili, ginger, and salt with 3 Tbsp of the olive oil in a food processor fitted with a metal blade. Process until a paste forms. Transfer to a large bowl. Put 2 Tbsp of the paste in a small bowl and stir in the lime juice to make the cilantro sauce. Cover and set aside.

Stir the curry powder into the rest of the paste, add the steak and coat well. Cover and marinate at room temp for about 20 min.

Cut the red onion into wedges and separate the wedges and thread beef and onion onto skewers. Brush a grill pan with the oil. Preheat grill pan and grill the kebabs for 8-10 minutes turning the skewers every 2 minutes. Serve with the cilantro sauce and bread. Serves 4.

Steak Filets with Peppercorn Mustard Sauce

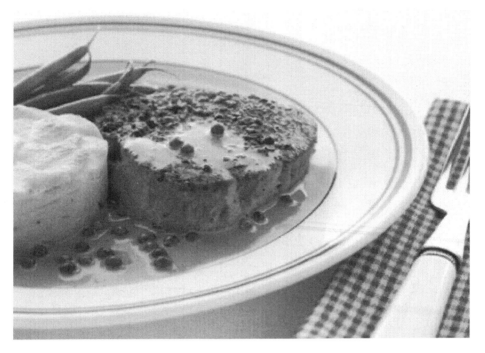

This meal is a simple and easy way to prepare a steak, but elegant enough for company too. Prepare this next time you have special guests, and you will be sure to please.

As long as it's grass-fed, red meat is not only very good for you, but it's a good idea to try to eat it twice a week or so—your body needs the vitamins and minerals that it contains. If you are an athlete, red meat provides vital building materials for your muscles—especially after hard workouts or athletic competition.

Peppercorns stimulate the taste buds and help to increase hydrochloric acid secretion in the stomach, which improves digestion of proteins, making them the perfect companion for steak. Peppercorns also have antioxidant and antibacterial effects. And while the outer layer of the peppercorn is working to help you digest your meal, it is also stimulating the breakdown of fat cells, keeping you slim and giving you energy to burn.

Maximize Your Flat Belly Journey: Get Powerful Fat Loss Secrets From Key Food And Fitness Experts.
http://velocityhousepresents.com/FlatBellyKitchen

Pepper is an excellent source of manganese, a very good source of iron and vitamin K, and a good source of dietary fiber.

Ingredients

- 4 (4 oz) grass-fed beef tenderloin filets (1½ inches thick)
- Sea salt, coarsely ground
- 2 Tbsp multi-colored, black or green peppercorns
- 4 Tbsp grass-fed organic butter
- ¼ cup minced shallots
- ½ cup dry red wine
- ½ cup organic beef broth
- ¼ cup Dijon mustard

Directions

Crush 1 Tbsp of the peppercorns with a rolling pin, and press salt and pepper into steaks. Heat butter in cast-iron skillet on medium high heat. Add steaks, turn heat to high and sear on both sides. Lower heat back to medium and cook 2-4 minutes on each side, depending on how well you like your steaks. DON'T OVERCOOK.

Remove steaks from pan; add shallots to pan, and sauté for 30 seconds. Add wine, cook for another 10 seconds or so. Add broth, mustard and the remaining tablespoon or so of the peppercorns, and stir well. Spoon sauce over steaks and serve. Enjoy with a tossed baby greens salad. Serves 2-4.

Stuffed Quinoa Peppers

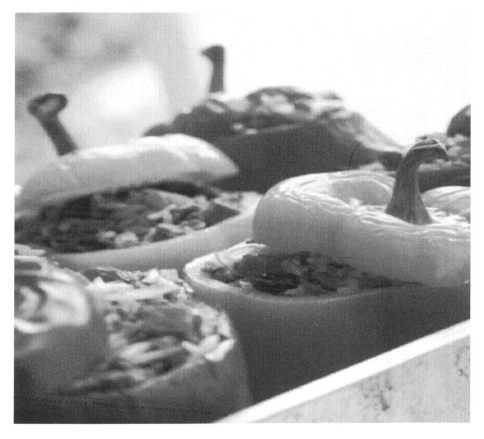

Quinoa is making a big appearance in grocery stores and restaurants these days—often as a substitute for rice—in pilafs, salads, or stuffings.

Quinoa is not actually a grain, but a seed that is full of high-energy nutrition. Quinoa is gluten-free, and a very good low glycemic carbohydrate source, rich in manganese, magnesium, calcium, copper, iron, phosphorus, vitamin E, and several B vitamins.

The protein in quinoa is superb. In fact, it contains an almost perfect balance of all 8 essential amino acids, to make it a complete protein source.

Cooked quinoa is excellent in casseroles and soups, stews, stir-fries, pilafs, or cold in salads. The seeds can be cooked in about 15 minutes. You can use quinoa to substitute for rice in most dishes. Quinoa comes in the 'traditional' white or tan color, red, which is a reddish-brown with a slightly richer flavor, and black. Black quinoa has a rich, nutty flavor and stays crunchier and firmer after cooking.

Ingredients
- 1 lb of grass-fed ground beef
- 4 red, yellow or green bell peppers, sliced in half, seeds and ribs removed
- 1 medium red onion, chopped
- 2-3 cloves of garlic, minced
- 1 small zucchini, diced
- ½ lb of fresh mushrooms, sliced, any variety
- 1-2 tsp of dried or fresh oregano (use double the amount if fresh)
- 1-2 tsp of dried or fresh basil (use double if fresh)
- 1 small can of organic, chopped tomatoes or 3 fresh Roma tomatoes, chopped
- Hot pepper flakes, to taste
- Sea salt, to taste
- 3-4 cups cooked quinoa
- Handful of chopped fresh parsley
- Several slices of your favorite grass-fed cheese, optional

Directions
Heat oven to 350 degrees F.
Wash peppers, remove stems and seeds, and cut in half from top to bottom. Place in a small (8"x 8" or 8" x 10") baking dish with sides.

In a frying pan over medium heat, cook beef until no longer pink, add in the onion, garlic, zucchini, mushrooms, oregano, basil, salt and pepper flakes.

Cook and stir about 5 minutes. Add in tomatoes and quinoa, and cook a few more minutes until most of the liquid is absorbed. Spoon meat mixture into the pepper "cups" and bake in oven, covered with foil for about 20-30 minutes.

Add cheese slices on top of peppers when there is about 5 minutes of cooking time left. Generously sprinkle parsley over peppers and serve. Serves 4.

Zesty Shish Kabobs

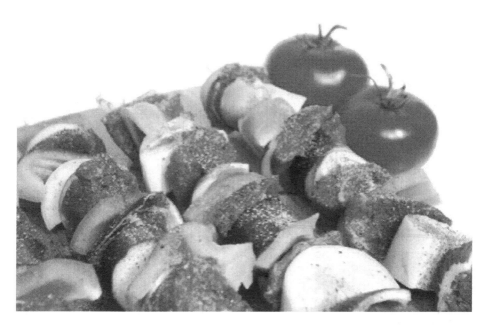

These are always a favorite at my house. You can use a specific 'kabob' cut of meat, or just buy a decent steak cut, like tenderloin, ribeye, or sirloin. For lamb, use leg or shoulder cut; for pork, the tenderloin or loin cuts work best, and for chicken, either boneless, skinless breast meat or thigh meat make tasty kabobs. And of course, always choose naturally raised, grass-fed, organic, and free-range meats if possible.

The bell peppers in this recipe contain large amounts of vitamin C and other antioxidants, and the more colorful ones (red, orange and yellow) not only make the shish kabob more appetizing, but they contain the most antioxidants as well. Use organic peppers if possible, as the conventionally grown versions are highly sprayed with pesticides.

Onions are an unsung and overlooked super food. They are often avoided because some varieties have a strong odor and taste. While lots of people avoid onions because they fear having bad breath, their awesome health benefits make up for that!

Onions contain some very strong cancer-fighting enzymes that lower the risk of prostate, esophageal, laryngeal, stomach, colorectal and ovarian cancers and also reduce the risk of dying from a heart attack.

Onions have super antioxidant power, especially the purple or red-skinned ones. The key antioxidant is quercetin, which acts as a natural antihistamine, reducing allergy attacks, inflammation and asthma. Quercetin and the vitamin C in onions act together to boost the immune system, and protect against colds and flu as well. The anti-inflammatory benefits help reduce the soreness and stiffness of arthritis and other inflammatory diseases. And onions, especially a sweet onion, develop a mellow, caramel-like sweetness when grilled that is hard to resist.

And don't forget the mushrooms! Mushrooms contain rich amounts of riboflavin, niacin, and selenium. They also contain chemicals that block excess estrogen production in men and women (which results in weight gain and 'manboobs'). They also boost natural testosterone, which is beneficial for both men and women, to help with building lean muscle, as well as increasing your fat burning potential.

While the fresh pineapple adds a delicious touch of sweet and tangy flavor, it also has beneficial enzymes in it that help digestion and absorption of the delicious nutrients in this dish.

Shish Kabob Ingredients
- 2 lbs beef, lamb, pork or chicken, cut into 1-1 ½ " cubes
- ½ lb of Baby Bella mushrooms or plain button mushrooms
- 1 large or 2 small sweet red onions or Vidalia onions, quartered
- 1 medium zucchini or summer squash cut into thick slices and cut in half
- 1 fresh pineapple cut in thick slices
- 1 each—green, yellow and red peppers, quartered and cut into 1" slices

Marinade
- 1 cup of soy sauce
- 3 Tbsp of honey
- Juice of 1 lime
- 1-2 cloves garlic, minced
- Freshly grated ginger root
- Couple shots of Tabasco or a few sprinkles of hot pepper flakes

Directions

Mix up marinade in glass bowl. Cut up meat and vegetables and place all *except the pineapple* (don't put pineapple in the marinade, it has natural enzymes in it that will turn your meat into MUSH) into the marinade.

Marinate for 1-4 hours or overnight for extra flavor.

Thread meat onto skewers and thread vegetables and pineapple onto separate skewers. (This prevents the vegetables from getting overcooked, as they cook quickly). On a grill over medium heat, grill meat and vegetables. Turn occasionally until evenly browned.

Delicious served with quinoa or alone. Serves 4.

Mike's Healthy Grilled Sardine Melt

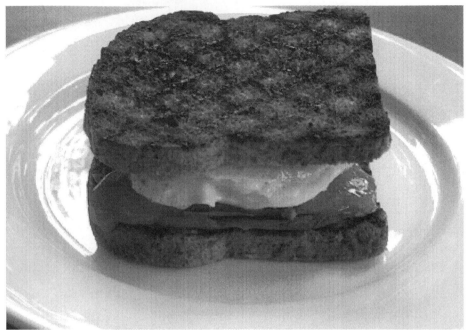

Photo courtesy Chef Ted Wood

While some of you less adventurous folks may turn up your nose at this recipe, you may be in for a surprise, as it is really quite delicious, filling and extremely good for you!

Sardines provide more calcium and phosphorus than milk, more protein than steak, more potassium than bananas, and more iron than cooked spinach. In addition, they are a valuable source of the nutrient CoQ10, which is highly beneficial in strengthening the heart muscle and increasing energy.

Sardines are a great, high omega 3 alternative, free of the worries of toxins and mercury inherent in tuna, swordfish, and other larger fish. If you have never considered sardines, or if you run away screaming from them, it's time to re-consider. They really are delicious—and very good for you too!

Sardines are a great choice for a quick, healthy meal or snack, full of lots of satisfying, muscle building protein; high in über-healthy, omega 3 fats, and low in mercury and other toxins.

Here is Mike's favorite protein-packed sandwich recipe:

Ingredients
- 1 can of sardines
- 1 whole egg cooked over-easy
- 2 slices of sprouted-grain Ezekiel bread (if you are feeling adventurous, try the raisin Ezekiel bread), or gluten-free whole-grain bread
- Grainy mustard
- 1 slice of grass-fed organic cheddar cheese
- Extra virgin olive oil, or pasture-raised butter to spread on the bread
- Arugula, fresh basil, and sliced tomatoes (optional)

Directions
Stack the cheese, sardines, egg and basil on the bread (with outsides brushed with extra virgin olive oil butter), and then grill this sandwich just like a grilled cheese sandwich.

Add arugula and fresh tomato when finished grilling.

This sandwich is great tasting! It's actually very good with sprouted-grain raisin bread for a taste contrast—as weird as that may sound—the sweetness of the raisins goes well with the sardines, egg, arugula and mustard. This is a filling sandwich and makes a great meal. Serves 1-2.

Easy Sweet And Spicy Salmon

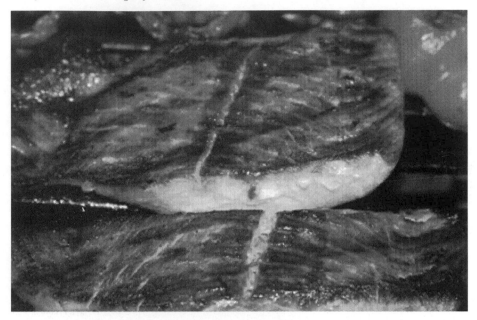

Salmon has a well-earned reputation as a health food because of its high omega 3 fatty acid content. A 4 ounce serving of wild caught salmon has 2 grams of omega 3 fats, which is more than the average adult (in the U.S.) gets in their diet in several days.

Omega 3 fats decrease your risk of heart attacks, strokes, arrhythmias, high blood pressure, and high triglycerides in the blood. Frequent consumption of salmon also decreases inflammation, helps cell membranes function better, prevents diabetes, and protects the brain.

Scientists consider DHA to be the most important fat for the human brain, and the high concentration of this fat in wild caught salmon decreases the risk of depression, hostility, and age-related forgetfulness. There is also an association between IQ and omega 3 intake, making salmon truly a 'brain superfood'.

If you would like quick and easy ways to get more salmon in your diet, this quick, easy and most importantly, delicious, recipe is for you. The sweetness of the maple syrup combines with the tanginess of the lime juice, and the heat of the pepper flakes to make a delicious, mouthwatering—but simple dish.

There are lots of different types of salmon: there's wild sockeye salmon with its deep pink flesh—my favorite and the most nutritious; king salmon—more mild tasting, but higher in good fats; keta salmon, Chinook, and chum salmon to name just a few.

You can adjust the ingredients in this recipe for virtually any amount of salmon. You—and everyone else—will love it!

Ingredients

- One or more pieces of fresh, wild caught salmon, any size—4 ounces to 1 lb or more.
- 1-2 Tbsp butter
- ¼ cup real maple syrup
- Juice of 1 lime
- Hot pepper flakes

Directions

Turn broiler on high and heat up. Move shelf to about 6 inches away from heat source. Place a small pat of butter on each piece or brush top of salmon with melted butter for best browning. Broil skin side down, 8-10 minutes, depending on the size and thickness of the salmon. Salmon can be eaten with the center still translucent and darker pink, or can be more well-done and opaque all the way through. Just be careful not to cook it for too long or it gets very dry. This fish can also be cooked on the grill over medium heat.

Remove fish from heat about 1-2 minutes before it looks done (it will cook a bit more after it is out). Don't overcook.

While fish is cooking, mix maple syrup, lime juice, and hot pepper flakes. (Go easy on the pepper, it can add a lot of heat!) When fish is done cooking, pour mixture over hot salmon and enjoy with a baked sweet potato and organic baby greens salad. Serves 2 or more.

Maximize Your Flat Belly Journey: Get Powerful Fat Loss Secrets From Key Food And Fitness Experts.
http://velocityhousepresents.com/FlatBellyKitchen

Salmon Patties

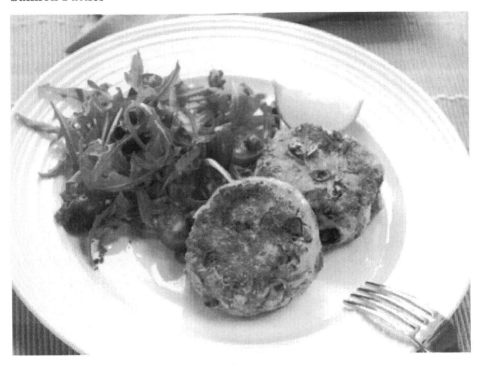

I make these salmon patties using canned wild red sockeye salmon. The wild caught, high omega 3, sockeye salmon comes from a company called Vital Choice. The bright red color means the salmon is not only full of flavor, but also a generous amount of omega 3's, and carotene antioxidants.

The flesh of salmon can range in color from pink to red to orange with some varieties richer in important omega 3 fatty acids than others. Chinook and sock- eye are fattier fish than pink and chum salmon, and contain greater amounts of healthy omega 3 fatty acids.

While salmon gets a lot of attention for being rich in omega 3 fatty acids, it also has other unique nutritional properties that are equally important. Salmon contains short protein molecules called peptides that possess significant anti-inflammatory properties.

Salmon also provides important amounts of the antioxidant amino acid taurine. Salmon is an excellent source of omega 3 fatty acids, vitamin D, and immune-supportive selenium. It is also a very good source of muscle-building protein, and heart-healthy B vitamins: niacin, B6 and B12; as well as a good source of energy-producing phosphorus and magnesium.

Since I like to spice things up a bit, I added some red pepper flakes and Frank's Redhot sauce to it. Cayenne and hot peppers actually raise the metabolism, fight inflammation, and protect the heart and blood vessels. The capsaicin in the hot pepper helps to burn fat, so besides the taste, it does great things for your body! Measurements are all approximate, so adjust the seasonings to your own taste.

Ingredients
- 2 cans (6.35oz) of wild caught sockeye salmon, un-drained
- 2 organic, free range eggs, beaten
- 1 tsp dill
- ½ cup gluten-free bread crumbs (or throw two slices of gluten-free or Ezekiel bread in your food processor and mix. Viola! Bread crumbs.)
- 1-2 tsp of Frank's Redhot sauce, to taste
- Juice of one lemon or lime
- 6-8 green onions, chopped
- Handful of parsley, minced
- ½ tsp of garlic powder or 1 garlic clove, minced
- Sea salt and pepper to taste
- 2 or more Tbsp of coconut oil and/or grass-fed butter, or any combination of oils.

Directions
Mix all ingredients except oil and ¼ cup of the flour/breadcrumb mixture in a glass bowl with a fork. I let the salmon mixture remain pretty chunky, as long as it will stick together.

Heat an iron skillet or frying pan over medium heat with the oil/butter. By hand, form small patties of the salmon mixture, dredge in flour, and place in pan.

Cook until golden brown about 5-6 minutes on each side. (Careful flipping the patties, they tend to fall apart easily). Serve with lemon wedges, hot sauce or plain organic yogurt. Serves 4.

Maximize Your Flat Belly Journey: Get Powerful Fat Loss Secrets From Key Food And Fitness Experts.
http://velocityhousepresents.com/FlatBellyKitchen

Alaskan Halibut or Cod with Butter Lime-Cilantro Sauce

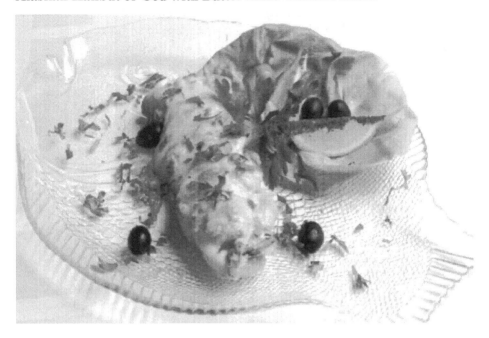

This recipe is adapted from my friends at Vital Choice Wild Seafood. They offer the best in fresh, wild caught, sustainable seafood, high in omega 3's. You won't find anything better!

Ingredients

- Four (6 oz each) halibut, or wild caught sablefish or cod • 3 Tbsp fresh lime juice
- 3 cloves garlic, coarsely chopped
- 1/2 cup chopped fresh cilantro
- 2 Tbsp butter
- 1 -2 Tbsp extra virgin olive oil or macadamia nut oil • Sea salt and coarse ground pepper

Directions

If you are grilling the fish, prepare the coals and oil the grate.

If you are broiling the fish, brush a broiler pan lightly with oil or butter. Brush the fish with about half of the lime juice, sprinkle with salt and pepper, and set aside for 20 or so minutes.

Meanwhile, melt the butter and extra virgin olive oil in a small pan over low heat. Add garlic and sauté until fragrant, about 3 minutes. Add the cilantro and the rest of the lime juice and stir for 1 minute. Remove from heat and cover.

Place fish on pre-heated grill over a medium high fire OR under a broiler. Grill or broil until just opaque in the center and flaky, about 4 to 5 minutes per side. Baste once with the oil-butter-cilantro-lime sauce, about one minute before the end of cooking.

Remove the fillets to a serving plate, pour the remaining sauce over them, and serve. Serves 4.

Maximize Your Flat Belly Journey: Get Powerful Fat Loss Secrets From Key Food And Fitness Experts.
http://velocityhousepresents.com/FlatBellyKitchen

Easy Chicken and Veggies in Foil Packets

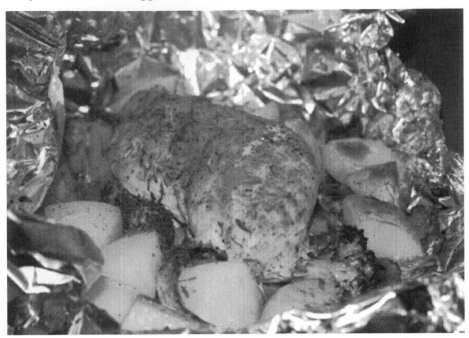

Cooking in foil packets is the basis for a great, quick and easy meal. Once you get the hang of it, you will find there are infinite variations—the only limit is your imagination!

Try substituting fish instead of the chicken, along with whatever veggies are in season at the time. You can use the oven, a charcoal or gas grill. If grilling, place packets away from direct heat so they do not overcook. I have even used this recipe a few times when camping as well, and it works beautifully on a grate over a fire too.

Potatoes are a delicious addition to this recipe. They soak up all the delicious juices of the other foods and spices. If you would like to use potatoes, cut them up in small pieces or slices, so they can cook thoroughly, otherwise the potatoes will take much longer to cook than the other vegetables.

Fresh or dried herbs and spices have huge amounts of concentrated antioxidants and nutrients, so try different combinations for a different taste sensation. And always be generous with the garlic too!

Ingredients

- 2 lbs skinless, boneless chicken breasts, sliced thin; or boneless, skinless thighs
- 1 red or white onion, sliced
- ½ lb fresh green beans, asparagus, sliced fresh zucchini, summer squash, etc.
- 2-4 white or sweet potatoes, quartered and sliced in ¼" or less thick pieces
- 2-4 Tbsp grass-fed butter, or extra virgin olive oil
- 1-2 cloves minced garlic
- 1 tsp (or more) oregano, basil, thyme, rosemary or other herbs; fresh or dried
- Sea salt, pepper
- Foil sheets, approximately 12" x 10"

Directions

Heat oven to 350-375 degrees F, or grill at medium heat.

Place a serving of meat in middle of foil sheet, spread vegetables on top, drizzle with extra virgin olive oil or a small chunk of grass-fed butter, season with garlic, herbs, salt and pepper, and wrap in a rectangular shaped package, bringing edges of foil together on top and sides and folding tightly a couple of times to seal in juices.

Place packets on a cookie sheet or shallow baking pan and bake in oven for about 30-40 minutes or until meat is cooked and vegetables are tender. If cooking on a grill, cook over medium-high heat, and place packets away from direct heat source. If cooking over a fire, wait until fire has died down some, and coals are glowing red.

For fish, shorten cooking time to about 20 minutes or less, as fish usually cooks quicker, depending on the size and type. Try wild caught salmon, cod or tilapia. Serves 4.

Healthy Chicken Cutlets

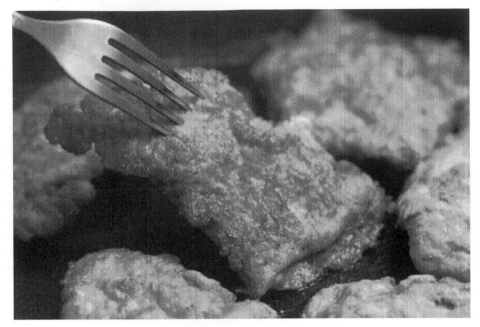

A far, far healthier alternative to the chicken tenders you would get at a restaurant, and the health benefits of the oregano in this recipe go way beyond the taste.

The crunchy crust of this chicken is seasoned with oregano. This delicious herb contains an active ingredient called rosmarinic acid, a very potent antioxidant that also has powerful antiviral, antibacterial, and antifungal properties.

Use a generous amount of fresh oregano, if you can get it, for the very best flavor. However, dried oregano works just as well, and the flavor is a bit more concentrated, so use less if dried.

The best oil to cook this chicken in is coconut oil. While it's delicate, it will not add a coconut flavor to the food, and it has the ability of maintaining its stability when heated, unlike olive oil.

Canola oil and other vegetable oils are highly processed oils (often genetically modified as well), full of inflammatory compounds. These oils become even more unhealthy when heated to high temperatures while cooking.

Ingredients
- 2 lbs of boneless, skinless chicken breasts or boneless, skinless thighs
- 2-3 eggs, beaten, in shallow dish
- 1 cup rice flour, coconut flour, or a mixture of both
- Sea salt and pepper
- 2 tsp garlic powder
- 3 Tbsp finely minced fresh parsley
- 1 tsp dried or fresh oregano (if fresh, minced)
- 3-4 Tbsp virgin coconut oil

Directions
Heat oven to 375 degrees F. Add dry seasoning and herbs to flour mixture. If using whole chicken breasts, slice in half to make thinner cutlets. You may pound these out with a meat pounder for added thinness, if you would like, but it is not necessary.

Dip each piece of chicken in the beaten egg, then dredge in breadcrumb mixture. Drizzle extra virgin olive oil on shallow cooking pans, and place chicken in pans. Cook in oven for about 10 minutes on one side, turn over then cook another 6-8 minutes, until golden brown and crispy. Serves 4.

Note: These make great leftovers and are delicious hot or cold. The cold leftovers are great sliced and added to a salad full of fresh veggies for a healthy, satisfying lunch.

Jerk Chicken With Pineapple Salsa

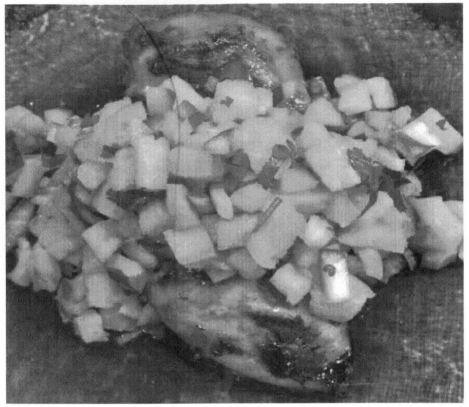

Photo courtesy of http://healthyandgourmet.blogspot.com

This chicken is best cooked on the grill, but can also be cooked in a pan on the stove with butter to brown the chicken. You can use pre-packaged jerk seasoning, or make your own (recipe included). Jerk seasoning is a spicy, sweet seasoning that Jamaicans use often in cooking. It can be found either wet or as a dry rub. The dry rub is the easiest to use, but either works.

Pineapple salsa makes a cool, sweet, and spicy-hot accompaniment to the chicken.

Pineapples are nutritionally packed, high fiber fruit, high in the enzyme bromelain, and the antioxidant vitamin C. Bromelain is a natural anti-inflammatory that is not only good for digestion, but encourages healing as well.

And don't forget, the hot peppers in this recipe will boost metabolism and burn fat too!

Ingredients
- 2 lbs of free-range chicken breasts, thighs or a whole cut up chicken
- 2 Tbsp of jerk seasoning (see recipe at bottom if you want to make it from scratch)

Pineapple Salsa
- 1 fresh pineapple, skinned, cored and diced in small pieces
- ¼ cup fresh cilantro
- 1 small red onion
- 1 small Roma tomato, finely chopped
- 1 jalapeño, de-seeded and de-ribbed (handle carefully and wash hands after cutting!)
- Juice of ½ fresh squeezed lime

Directions
Rub jerk seasoning generously over chicken and cook over medium heat on grill or in pan with extra virgin olive oil. Turn and cook until golden brown and not pink inside.

While chicken is cooking, chop up ingredients for pineapple salsa, and mix together with the fresh squeezed lime. Serve with the cooked chicken. Serves 4 or so.

Mix together all the ingredients. This salsa is great and refreshing and can be used on fish, chicken, and pork for a zippy, delicious seasoning.

Jerk Seasoning
- 1 Tbsp onion flakes
- 2 tsp ground thyme
- 1 tsp ground allspice
- 1/4 tsp ground cinnamon
- 1 tsp black pepper
- 1 tsp cayenne pepper
- 1 Tbsp onion powder
- 2 tsp sea salt

Maximize Your Flat Belly Journey: Get Powerful Fat Loss Secrets From Key Food And Fitness Experts.
http://velocityhousepresents.com/FlatBellyKitchen

- 1/4 tsp ground nutmeg
- 2 tsp sugar

Turkey or Chicken Meatballs

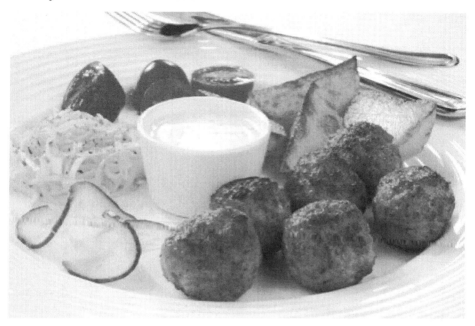

I love these and you will too! They're a great source of healthy protein. I like to add a generous amount of fresh garlic to maximize the nutrition in this recipe.

Ingredients
- 1 lb ground free-range organic turkey or chicken • 1 raw egg
- 1 onion, minced
- 2-4 cloves garlic, minced
- 1 tsp sea salt or so, to taste
- 1 slice gluten-free bread, blended into crumbs in a food processor, 1/2 cup
- oatmeal, 1/2 cup ground flax seeds, or any combination of these • 1-2 tsp of oregano
- 2 Tbsp of extra virgin olive oil

Directions
Heat oven to 375 degrees F. Drizzle extra virgin olive oil on cookie sheets (with sides) or a shallow baking pan.

In a big bowl, combine all remaining ingredients. Mix with clean hands or large wooden spoon. Roll into 1 ½" sized balls, and place on the baking sheet in oven. Cook for about 10 minutes or so, turn (or roll) and cook another ten minutes, for a total of about 20 minutes. Done when outside is golden brown and inside is no longer pink.

Serve with your favorite organic spaghetti sauce and steamed spaghetti squash, or just eat plain alongside a salad. I have even had cold leftover meatballs (which are delicious by the way!) on Caesar salads for healthy lunch. Serves 4.

These are a great high protein snack too!

Warm Asian Steak Salad

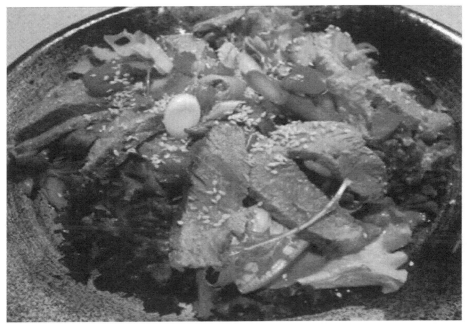

Photo courtesy of Just Jan, http://janandrussroundozagain-janandruss.blogspot.com

This salad contains fresh ginger in the dressing. I love its fresh, zingy flavor. But there are more reasons to enjoy ginger than just flavor. Ginger is an incredible superfood that does many, many good things for your body, including helping you burn fat efficiently by speeding up your metabolism.

Ginger actually promotes normal levels of both LDL ("bad") cholesterol and triglycerides. It's a delicious way to get these unhealthy fats down to manageable levels.

Eating ginger every day can give you a real antioxidant boost. That's because ginger contains 12 antioxidant compounds more powerful than vitamin E! And, studies show that ginger soothes the body's inflammatory response and promotes healthy circulation as well.

Some of ginger's other benefits are well known too. You may already know that ginger is great for nausea and motion sickness—and works as well or better than some medications.

Maximize Your Flat Belly Journey: Get Powerful Fat Loss Secrets From Key Food And Fitness Experts.
http://velocityhousepresents.com/FlatBellyKitchen

Ginger is an excellent digestive aid as well. It really helps get your digestive system moving. And ginger's zippy flavor also jumpstarts your metabolism by making you more energetic and burn more calories.

Salad Ingredients
- 3/4 lb grass-fed sirloin, skirt or tri-tip steak
- Mixed organic greens (romaine, arugula, red leaf, etc.)
- 10-12 stalks of asparagus trimmed, cooked slightly and cut in 1 inch pieces
- 1 sweet red pepper, cut in thin strips
- ½ seedless cucumber, thinly sliced
- 3 green onions thinly sliced
- Handful of chopped fresh cilantro
- Chopped tomato
- Toasted sesame seeds or peanuts

Dressing Ingredients
- ½ cup orange juice
- ½ Tbsp fresh ginger minced or grated
- ½ Tbsp rice wine vinegar
- 2 cloves garlic, smashed and minced
- 2 tsp soy sauce
- 2 tsp sesame oil
- 2 tsp honey
- 1 tsp extra virgin olive oil
- 1 dash hot pepper sauce (optional)

Directions
Whisk together dressing ingredients. Pour ¼ cup of dressing over steak in a shallow glass dish, turning to coat. Reserve remaining dressing. Grill steak about 3-4 minutes per side (if steak is about 1" thick). Let steak rest for a few minutes before carving. Slice thinly on the diagonal.

In a serving dish, toss reserved dressing with salad greens, asparagus, red pepper, cucumber, green onions and coriander. Add steak to top of salad and garnish with sesame seeds or peanuts, and serve. Serves 4.

Salad Niçoise

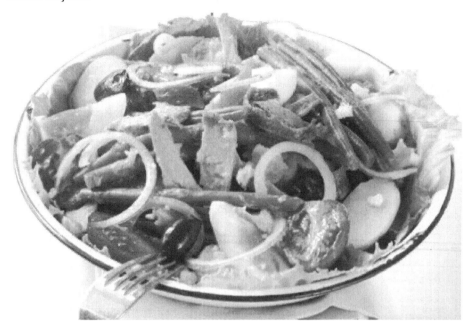

High in protein, healthy fats and fiber, this salad Niçoise makes a satisfying and incredibly healthy meal. You can make it hours before, and add the tuna and dressing just before serving. Substitute tuna with canned or leftover wild salmon, or any other piece of cooked fish you may have left over.

Dark green leafy salad greens and vegetables are alkalizing foods. The American Journal of Clinical Nutrition says alkalizing diets rich in leafy, raw vegetables improve bone density and increase growth hormones. I really like the baby arugula with its sharp, slightly bitter taste. Arugula is a member of the cabbage family, which makes it an excellent fat burning, cancer-fighting food, and an excellent source of vitamins A and C, folic acid, calcium, manganese, and magnesium, as well as potassium, iron, zinc, riboflavin, and copper.

Salads become a prebiotic in your gut. Prebiotics are non-digestible high fiber foods that stimulate growth of healthy gut bacteria, probiotics. By having a good supply of probiotics in the gut, you boost your immune system, and absorb nutrients from food better.

Maximize Your Flat Belly Journey: Get Powerful Fat Loss Secrets From Key Food And Fitness Experts.
http://velocityhousepresents.com/FlatBellyKitchen

And don't be afraid of the potatoes. An occasional potato will not hurt your efforts to stay lean, especially when it is combined with other fiber rich vegetables, healthy fats, and good quality protein. Potatoes, especially organic ones, are rich in nutrients.

Salad Ingredients
- 2 or 3 big handfuls of baby greens, chopped red leaf lettuce or romaine
- 2 handfuls of baby arugula
- 2-3 new red potatoes, quartered
- ½ lb or so fresh or frozen organic green beans or asparagus
- 4 eggs hard-boiled, quartered
- 2 large or 3 smaller ripe tomatoes, chopped
- 1/3 cup kalamata or Greek olives
- ½ large red onion sliced thinly
- Handful of chopped parsley
- 1 small can of tuna or wild salmon (drained), or equal amount of cooked fish
- Capers for garnish

Dressing Ingredients
- 1-2 garlic cloves, smashed and minced
- 1 small shallot, minced
- ½ cup extra virgin olive oil
- ¼ cup balsamic vinegar or fresh lemon juice
- ½ tsp Dijon mustard
- Sea salt and pepper to taste

Directions
Steam green beans or asparagus lightly until tender crisp and then cool under cold water. Boil potatoes and cool. Whisk together ingredients for dressing.

On a large plate or shallow bowl, place greens on bottom, and arrange potatoes, green beans, eggs, tomatoes, olives and tuna in separate sections on top of greens. Drizzle with dressing and garnish with capers. Serves 2-4.

Chicken Fiesta Salad with Lime Cilantro Vinaigrette

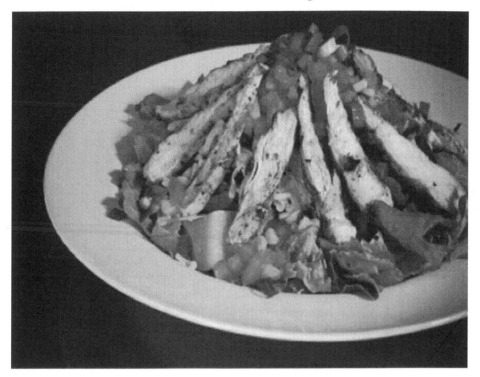

Ever feel sometimes you just need the maximum amount of nutrition in one meal? Don't fresh, raw veggies, and flavor that bursts in your mouth sound good? Something so satisfyingly different, delicious, and delightful that you serve it when you have company?

This is the salad that answers all those requirements.

Everything in this salad is absolutely packed with a massive amount of fat burning vitamins, minerals and phytochemicals! From the antioxidants, vitamin K, vitamin C and magnesium in the greens, the healthy fats in the avocado, the lycopene in the tomatoes, to the cancer-fighting natural chemicals in the tomatillo—it's all great for your body!

I always feel full of energy after eating this wonderful salad, and I love to make this when I have company over—it's a proven crowd pleaser. It's even better in the summer when so many of these ingredients are easy to find local-

201

ly, bursting with fresh-picked flavor. I am positive this will become one of your personal favorites too.

Dressing

- ¼ cup chopped shallots
- ¼ cup fresh lime juice (juice of 1 lime)
- ½ cup fresh cilantro chopped
- 2-3 cloves of finely minced garlic
- 1/3 cup extra virgin olive oil
- Sea salt and fresh ground pepper

Dressing Directions

Combine first four ingredients in medium bowl. Gradually whisk in oil. Season with sea salt and pepper.

Salad

- 3 cups of thinly sliced red leaf lettuce (preferably organic)
- 3 cups thinly sliced Napa cabbage
- 2-3 Roma tomatoes, seeded and chopped
- ½ roasted red bell pepper (you can usually find these already roasted in the store or see below on how to roast your own)
- ½ roasted yellow pepper
- Half (or more) firm avocado, peeled and diced
- ¼ cup minced red onion
- Half a can black beans, drained and rinsed
- 1 small jalapeno, de-seeded, de-ribbed and minced
- 2 small tomatillos, hulls removed and chopped (green Mexican tomatoes)
- ¼ cup toasted pumpkin seeds
- ½ cup crumbled queso anejo, or feta cheese (optional)
- 2-4 cooked chicken breasts, cooked and sliced in thin strips, or shredded with a fork
- (Grilled chicken tastes best for this recipe.)

Salad Directions

Combine salad ingredients in large bowl and toss in dressing just before serving. Place cut or shredded chicken on top. Serves 4-6.

To roast peppers: heat oven on 'broil'. Slice peppers in half; remove stem and seeds. Place skin side up on flat pan in oven near heat. Roast for 4-7 minutes until skin begins to turn black. Remove and cool. When cool, slide off blackened skin and slice peppers in thin strips.

Wine Country Chicken Salad

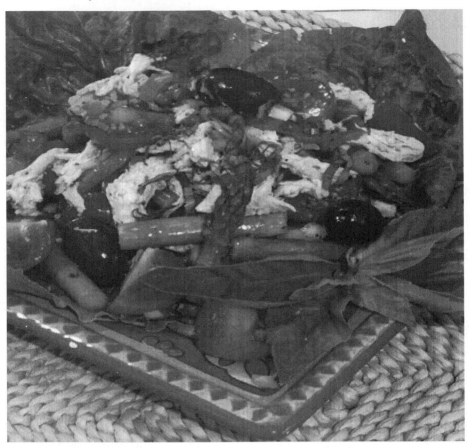

This recipe is one of my favorites, adapted from a recipe from the Robert Mondavi Winery in Napa Valley. It makes a perfect meal with high quality protein, good-for-you fats, and healthy greens loaded with antioxidants and fat burning power. And, it's beautiful looking too.

The dressing contains the fresh herbs, thyme and basil. Thyme and basil contain healthy volatile oils with well-documented health benefits. The oil in thyme, '*thymol*' can actually increase the amount of healthy fats in your cell membranes and other cell structures. When you eat omega 3 fats containing DHA (a very important part of omega 3's), thyme helps to get those healthy fats right where your body needs them. It even protects brain cells and decreases aging. So, thyme and omega 3 fats are a winning combination!

Thyme also contains a variety of flavonoids, including *apigenin, naringenin, luteolin,* and *thymonin*. These flavonoids increase thyme's antioxidant power, and combined with the manganese it contains, put thyme at the top of the list of powerful antioxidants.

Basil actually contains a substance that works like anti-inflammatory medication like ibuprofen. It provides relief for people with inflammatory health problems like arthritis or inflammatory bowel conditions.

The really interesting thing about both basil and thyme is their ability to kill certain bacteria and fungi. *Staphalococcus aureus (staph), Bacillus subtilis, Escherichia coli (e.coli),* and *Shigella sonnei* are some of the food-borne bacteria that these herbs can kill.

So you see, it makes very good sense to include thyme and basil in your recipes, especially for foods that are uncooked, such as salads. Adding generous amounts of fresh thyme and basil to your next vinaigrette will not only enhance the flavor of your fresh greens, but will help ensure that your fresh produce is safe to eat. Enjoy!

Salad
- 3 cups chicken stock or water
- 2 boneless skinless chicken breasts
- ½ lb pencil thin asparagus, cut into 2" pieces
- ½ cup Nicoise olives, pitted
- 10 cherry tomatoes, quartered
- 2 Tbsp capers, drained and rinsed
- 2 Tbsp finely chopped fresh basil
- Parmigiano-Reggiano, shaved or grated

Dressing
- ½ cup extra virgin olive oil
- 1 medium shallot minced
- 2 generous tsp finely chopped fresh thyme
- 1 Tbsp or more finely chopped fresh parsley

- ¼ cup fresh lemon juice (1 medium lemon)
- Sea salt and pepper to taste

Directions

In a deep medium-sized saucepan bring the stock or water to a simmer. Add the whole pieces of chicken and simmer for 10-12 minutes until tender. Cool chicken in the liquid, drain and shred the chicken by tearing into long thin pieces with forks. Set aside. Cook the asparagus for 3-4 minutes until tender but crisp. Drain and cool under cold water.

Add olives, tomatoes, capers, basil and pepper to the chicken and stir to combine.

Mix the ingredients for the dressing, and add to the salad mixture. Stir gently to combine. Arrange on a bed of organic baby greens, Bibb lettuce, or red leaf lettuce. Garnish with some Parmigiano-Reggiano (this is the Italian version of Parmesan cheese, it's usually raw and aged, and way tastier). Using a vegetable peeler, just peel a few thin pieces onto the salad.

This can be prepared up to 6 hours ahead of time and refrigerated. Add the dressing just prior to serving. Serves 2-4, depending on appetites.

A Healthier Mayonnaise

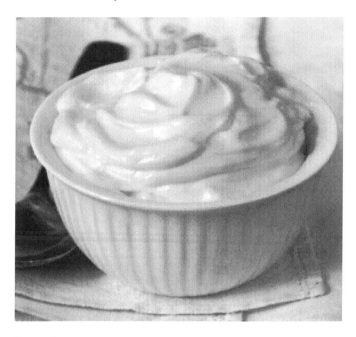

Ingredients
- 1 whole (fresh, organic) egg • 2 egg yolks
- 1 Tbsp Dijon mustard
- 1 Tbsp lemon juice
- Sea salt to taste
- 1⁄4 tsp white pepper or black pepper
- 2/3 cup Udo's Choice Oil or extra virgin olive oil

Directions
Combine the eggs, mustard, lemon juice, salt and white pepper in your blender or food processor. Then with the blender or food processor running on a low speed, start adding the oils very slowly. Start out with drops and then work up to about a small stream. It takes about 5 minutes to accomplish this, but the end result is worth it! Continue blending until all the oil is incorporated.

Makes about 11⁄2 cups. Refrigerate to thicken. Store in an airtight container for up to two weeks.

Maximize Your Flat Belly Journey: Get Powerful Fat Loss Secrets From Key Food And Fitness Experts.
http://velocityhousepresents.com/FlatBellyKitchen

Quinoa Tabouli Salad

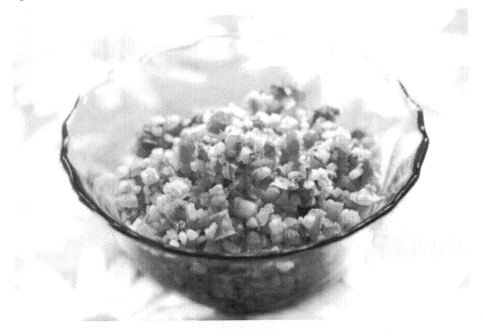

This Middle Eastern salad normally uses cracked wheat, but quinoa is a great, gluten-free healthy substitute. Since quinoa is not really a grain, but a low-gly- cemic, high protein seed—packed with antioxidants, nutrients and all the es- sential amino acids—it is definitely a better substitute!

Quinoa is high in protein, and it's a complete protein, containing all essential amino acids, especially the amino acid lysine, which is important to tissue growth and repair.

Quinoa also contains manganese, iron, copper and phosphorus along with antioxidants, B vitamins, and fiber, making it a great healthy food for everyone but especially anyone with migraine headaches, diabetes, and heart disease.
Eating quinoa will help migraines and headaches. How? Quinoa is a great source of magnesium, something that most of us are lacking enough of in our diets. Magnesium helps relax blood vessels, which helps to prevent the dilation and constriction of migraines.

Magnesium levels are also directly associated with blood pressure, so getting adequate amounts of magnesium in your diet will help to lower blood pressure and regulate your heartbeat. Quinoa is also a great source of riboflavin, a B vitamin necessary for proper energy production.

An excellent picnic food idea, it tastes great chilled or at room temperature, and won't spoil easily.

Ingredients
- 2 cups cooked quinoa, drained
- 1 organic cucumber, chopped
- 2 medium tomatoes, chopped
- 1 bunch green onions, (8) sliced
- ½ cup fresh chopped mint
- 2 cups fresh chopped parsley
- 2 cloves garlic, minced

Dressing
- ½ cup fresh lemon juice
- ¾ cup extra virgin olive oil
- Sea salt and freshly ground pepper, to taste

Directions
Cut up the vegetables for the salad, and toss with the dressing. This will have better flavor if allowed to soak up the dressing and flavors for an hour or more. Serve chilled or at room temperature. Serves 4-6.

Oriental Cabbage Salad

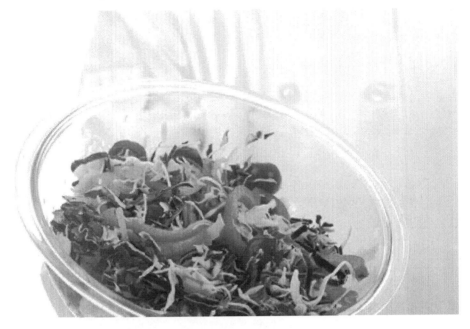

Cabbage belongs to the family of cruciferous vegetables, along with broccoli, cauliflower, Brussels sprouts, arugula, and kale. It contains a very unique phytonutrient called indole-3-carbinol (I3C). This unique plant nutrient blocks the adverse effects of certain types of chemicals known as xenoestrogens (or artificial estrogens) in our environment that cause the storage of extra abdominal fat, 'manboobs,' and other unwanted physical effects.

Xenoestrogens can mimic estrogen in the body and the excess estrogen can make you more prone to reproductive cancers such as prostate cancer in men, and breast and ovarian cancer in women.

Since xenoestrogens are found in so many things we encounter in our environment, on a daily basis, it is nearly impossible to avoid them completely. So, making sure you get plenty of this nutrient is a powerful way to fight against these estrogenic compounds, avoid belly fat, and protect yourself against cancer.

Cruciferous vegetables are also full of fiber and other cancer-fighting ingredients as well. This salad is a nice high fiber change to a regular lettuce salad.

Ingredients
- 1/2 regular green cabbage, shredded or sliced very thinly
- 1/4 red cabbage, shredded
- 1 carrot, shredded
- 4-6 green onions, chopped
- 1 sweet red bell pepper, slivered
- 1 apple, sliced and slivered
- 1/2 cup of slivered almonds
- 1 Tbsp toasted sesame seeds or black sesame seeds

Dressing
- 1/2 tsp of sesame oil
- 2 Tbsp of peanut oil
- 2-3 Tbsp rice wine vinegar
- Squirt of honey
- 1 Tbsp of fresh grated ginger
- Juice of half a lime
- Sea salt
- Hot pepper flakes, to taste

Directions
Add all ingredients to a glass bowl, add in dressing and mix!
Delicious with salmon or any other wild caught fish. This tastes even better the next day! Serves 4-6.

Maximize Your Flat Belly Journey: Get Powerful Fat Loss Secrets From Key Food And Fitness Experts.
http://velocityhousepresents.com/FlatBellyKitchen

Green Bean Salad

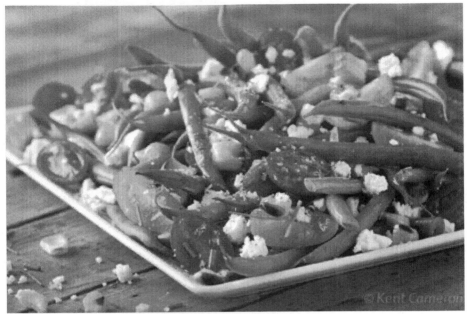

Recipe and Photo courtesy of Kent and Karen Cameron, afoodcentriclife.com

Green beans can be delicious and tender, or tough and woody, depending on where and when you get them. Obviously, they are best grown locally because they are usually the most tender and fresh.

Green beans are an excellent source of vitamin A and C, vitamin K and manganese, an important trace mineral. They also contain beta carotene, fiber, potassium, folate, and iron. On top of that, green beans are also a good source of magnesium, thiamin, riboflavin, copper, calcium, phosphorus, protein, omega 3 fatty acids and niacin.

One cup of green beans provides 25% of your vitamin K, which is as important as calcium for strong bones. Vitamins A and C fight free radicals in your body and help prevent cholesterol from building up in blood vessel walls. Magnesium and potassium help lower high blood pressure and work to calm you mentally and physically.

Commercially grown green beans from the grocery store are sprayed with a lot of pesticides, so buy organic and local whenever you can. This is best if you can prepare it ahead of time or at least save some as leftovers so the flavors can develop more and blend together.

This colorful green bean salad is a great side dish for grilled meat, poultry and fish. Serve chilled—it's great for hot weather entertaining, picnics and tailgating.

Ingredients
- 12 ounces baby green beans, ends trimmed
- Half pound cherry tomatoes in mixed colors, halved lengthwise
- 4-6 oz feta cheese, crumbled
- Salt and pepper, to taste, plus salt for boiling the green beans
- Fresh chopped basil, oregano, or chives

Vinaigrette
- 2/3 cup extra virgin olive oil
- Zest of one lemon
- ½ cup fresh squeezed lemon juice
- 2 Tbsp chopped fresh mint
- 1 large garlic clove, finely chopped
- 1/2 tsp kosher salt
- 1/4 tsp black pepper

Directions
Fill a large bowl with ice and cold water. Bring a large pot of water (4-5 quarts) to a boil and add a tablespoon of salt. Add green beans and cook for 4-5 minutes.

At 4 minutes, quickly toss one green bean into the ice water to test for doneness. They should be crisp-tender. When they reach that point, remove the beans from heat, drain off water, and place them immediately in the ice water to stop the cooking process and set the color.

After a few minutes in the ice water, drain the beans and allow them to dry. At this point you can refrigerate the green beans until you are ready to serve them. You can even cook them a day ahead.

When ready to serve, make the vinaigrette in separate bowl and mix by hand.

Add the greens, tomatoes, and cheese to a large bowl. Toss with a few table-spoons of the vinaigrette and season with salt and pepper to taste. Sprinkle on additional chopped fresh herbs if using. Serves 4-6.

Fresh Cucumber and Tomato Salad

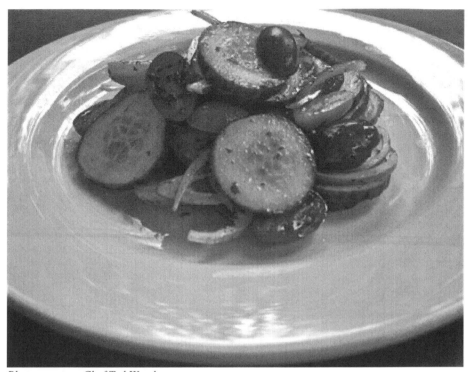

Photo courtesy Chef Ted Wood

This salad is, by far, the best in the summer when big luscious tomatoes are in season and full of flavor, and the cucumbers are fresh and tender.

Cucumbers don't seem to be the sexy new superfood topping all the lists lately, but this vegetable pulls its own weight in the nutrition and fat-burning category for sure! Cucumbers contain very valuable antioxidant, anti-inflammatory, and anti-cancer benefits.

While cucumbers are a great source of conventional nutrients including vitamin C, vitamin A, and manganese, they also contain numerous antioxidants, including quercetin, apigenin, luteolin, and kaempferol, and a substance called cucurbitacins.

Pharmaceutical companies are actively studying cucurbitacins—to develop new anti-cancer drugs. Cucurbitacins actually can block cancer cell development. Cucumbers also contain another ingredient, lignans, that fight cancer as well. When we eat lignans from vegetables, bacteria in our digestive tract convert them into substances that fight breast, ovarian, uterine, and prostate cancers.

Tomatoes add cancer-fighting lycopene, vitamins C and A, as well as antioxidants, and the herbs add even more powerful antioxidant properties as well.

And remember, all these antioxidants are not only really great for your health, but they also have great fat-burning power as well! Not to mention, this salad is naturally very low in calories, high in fiber and very filling.

Ingredients
* 2-3 fresh tomatoes, chopped in large pieces
* 3-4 smaller cucumbers or 2 larger ones, peeled and sliced
* (I sometimes use baby organic cucumbers and you can leave the skin on these)
* 1 sweet Vidalia or red onion, sliced and quartered
* Fresh oregano, thyme, or basil in any combination, chopped

Dressing Ingredients
* ¼ to ½ cup organic apple cider vinegar, or rice wine vinegar
* 1 tsp raw sugar
* ¼ cup extra virgin olive oil
* Sea salt and pepper to taste

Directions
Chop up vegetables and herbs and place in bowl. Pour dressing mix over the top and mix. This salad tastes better if you can prepare ahead of time and let it sit for a while, so the flavors all mix together better. Serves 2-4.

Cooked Greens and Herb Pesto

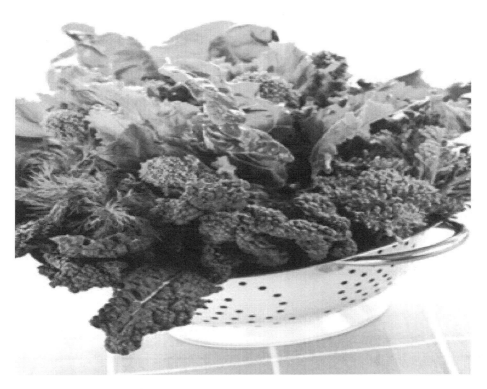

In this recipe, an assortment of greens is steamed then lightly drizzled with the pesto—extra virgin olive oil and a blend of cilantro, garlic, and parsley with lots of cumin. A squeeze of fresh lemon juice adds the perfect touch. This salad is good hot from the pan or at room temperature.

Collard greens, turnip greens, mustard greens, and kale belong to the same plant family as broccoli, Brussels sprouts, cabbage and cauliflower. Not only are these *cruciferous* vegetables great fat-burners, but they also protect your health and prevent cancer, by providing you with a very rich source of vita- mins, minerals and phytochemicals.

And here's another great fact about these superfood vegetables—did you know that certain chemicals like pesticides, herbicides and everyday house hold chemicals and cosmetics in our food and environment can mimic the female hormone estrogen?

"Xenoestrogens" as these chemicals are called, have a negative effect on men and women. Exposure to xenoestrogens can really mess up the hormone balance in both men and women. One of the things these estrogenic chemicals do is stimulate your body to store belly fat and, even worse, they encourage cancer growth.

Cruciferous vegetables contain unique phytonutrients such as indole-3-carbinol (I3C) that help to fight and block the effects of these estrogenic compounds. So you get healthier *and fight belly fat* when you eat them!

In addition, there are 10-15 compounds these leafy greens contain that have been proven effective against many cancers, including: stomach cancer, prostate cancer, colon cancer, breast cancer, and ovarian cancer.

These greens also contain large amounts of vitamin A, vitamin C, B6, manganese, calcium, copper, and potassium. These nutrients help reduce damage from inflammation, lower cholesterol, fight infections, and strengthen and renew collagen in the skin for a healthy youthful appearance.

In addition, the manganese helps with the production of sex hormones and protects the nervous system. It also helps to metabolize and utilize energy from protein and carbohydrates, making it the perfect fat-burning mineral.

Kale, collard greens, mustard and turnip green contain large amounts of bone-strengthening calcium, and when combined with vitamins A and K2 (a necessary nutrient for bone health) in grass-fed butter, it works to get calcium to where it is needed, strengthening bones and teeth.

There is absolutely no question that these cruciferous greens are one of the world's most powerful foods to burn fat and protect your health! Eat them as often as you can.

Herb Pesto
- 4 large garlic cloves
- Sea salt

- 1-2 good handfuls of parsley leaves
- 1 or 2 handfuls of cilantro leaves
- 3 Tbsp of extra virgin olive oil
- 2 tsp paprika
- 2 tsp ground cumin
- 1 lemon cut into wedges
- Handful of pine nuts (optional)

Greens

A couple of big bunches of greens in any combination, such as: kale, mustard, arugula, watercress, dandelion, chard, escarole, collard greens, organic spinach, etc. You can use one kind or mix a few together. If you like greens with a strong flavor, use mustard, collard, kale or dandelion greens. If you prefer a sweeter milder flavor, use chard and spinach.

Directions

Wash the greens well and cut away tough stems and chop in smaller pieces. Put the greens in a shallow pan with about a ¼ cup of water. Cover and steam until tender about 5-7 minutes. Drain off excess water.

In a food processor, add garlic, salt, parsley, cilantro and pine nuts, and process until finely chopped.

Gradually warm the extra virgin olive oil in a pan, with the paprika and cumin. When it begins to smell good, (1-2 minutes) add the garlic-herb mixture to the oil. Next add the greens and stir. Heat for a minute and pile into a dish. Garnish with lemon wedges. Serves 4-6.

Fresh Zucchini and Tomatoes with Basil

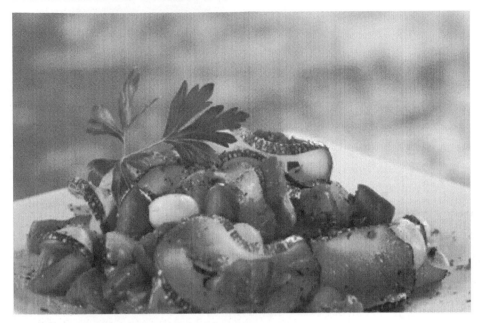

When zucchini and tomatoes are in season, nothing compares to the delicate nutty taste of fresh picked zucchini and the sweet, juicy tang of tomatoes. Finding both of these locally grown means that these vegetables are at their peak of flavor and nutrition.

Tomatoes are powerhouses of energy packed nutrition—full of lycopene and antioxidants, including vitamins A and C. Zucchini, or summer squash, as it may be called, is an excellent source of manganese and vitamin C, magnesium, vitamin A, fiber, potassium, folate, copper, riboflavin, and phosphorus.

The magnesium in zucchini is a relaxant for the body and the muscles, and also reduces the risk of heart attack and stroke. Together with potassium, magnesium reduces high blood pressure. Vitamin C and vitamin A are hearty antioxidants and help to prevent the buildup of cholesterol in the blood vessels, along with their fat burning capabilities.

Basil contains flavonoids and volatile oils which are uniquely health protecting. Basil actually provides protection against dangerous bacteria which can cause food poisoning, including: *Listeria, Staphs, E.coli* O:157:H7, and more.

Basil is also a very good source of vitamin A and magnesium, which improves blood flow and helps the heart beat more regularly. Basil contains iron, calcium, and plenty of potassium and vitamin C.

Note: The oils in basil are highly volatile; it is best to add the herb near the end of the cooking process, so it will retain its maximum essence and flavor.

Ingredients
- 2 Tbsp of extra virgin olive oil
- 1 lb or so of fresh, small zucchini, sliced thinly
- 1-2 cloves of garlic, crushed and minced
- 2-3 firm, medium to small tomatoes, chopped (Roma tomatoes are good for this)Sea salt
- Fresh ground pepper
- A handful of fresh basil, chopped
- Couple thin slices of prosciutto, chopped, (or nitrite-free cooked bacon)

Directions
Over medium heat, add extra virgin olive oil, zucchini, and garlic and cook for a couple of minutes until zucchini becomes slightly tender. Add tomatoes, salt and pepper and toss. Remove from heat and toss in prosciutto or bacon, and basil. Enjoy! For a protein packed meal, add this to scrambled eggs. Serves 4.

Maximize Your Flat Belly Journey: Get Powerful Fat Loss Secrets From Key Food And Fitness Experts.
http://velocityhousepresents.com/FlatBellyKitchen

Roasted Cauliflower

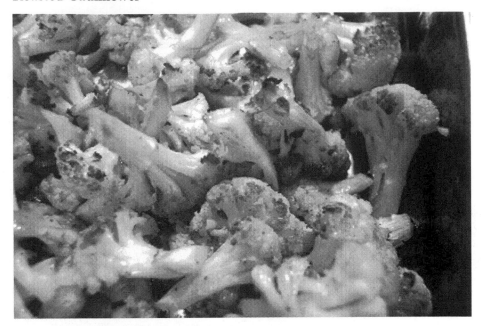

Here is another way to enjoy the healthy, fat-burning, high-fiber, cancer-fighting benefits of cauliflower. You will want to include cauliflower as a vegetable you eat on a regular basis to get some of the great health benefits it offers. Cruciferous vegetables, like cauliflower, broccoli, kale, Brussels sprouts and others should be included in your diet 3-5 times a week.

Cauliflower provides nutrients for three body systems that are directly tied to cancer: the detoxification system, the antioxidization system, and inflammatory system. Problems in any one of these three systems can lead to cancer, so protecting and optimizing these systems is vital to good health.

If you have never had roasted cauliflower before, you are in for a real treat. The roasting process along with real butter, gives it a nutty sweet flavor, unlike any other method of cooking. This is truly delicious!

<u>Ingredients</u>
- 1 head of cauliflower
- 2-3 cloves garlic, peeled and coarsely minced

- 1 lemon
- 2-4 Tbsp grass—fed butter
- Coarse salt and freshly ground black pepper
- Parmigiano-Reggiano cheese, grated (this is the Italian aged raw milk version of Parmesan cheese)

If you like, add smoked paprika or some fresh herbs like basil, oregano, thyme or rosemary for added fat-burning and nutritional benefits.

Directions

Preheat your oven to 400 degrees F. Cut the cauliflower into smaller florets and put in a single layer in a baking dish. Add minced garlic. Squeeze a lemon over the cauliflower florets and add some chunks of grass-fed butter.

Season with salt and pepper and any herbs you would like to add.

Bake for 20 to 25 minutes or until the cauliflower is just starting to brown. Sprinkle with Parmigiano-Reggiano or Parmesan cheese. Delicious and easy! Serves 4, give or take.

Roasted Brussels Sprouts with Bacon

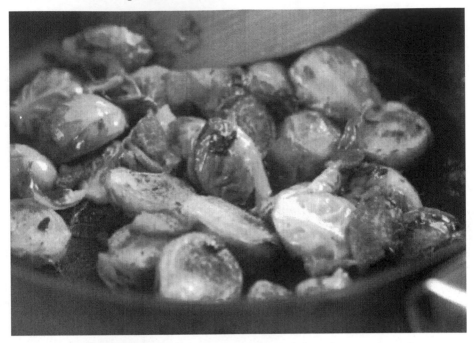

Even if you are an avowed Brussels sprouts hater, I am certain you will change your mind once you try this recipe. These caramelly-sweet, roasted Brussels sprouts with bacon will transform anyone into a Brussels sprouts lover!

Brussels sprouts are members of the auspicious cruciferous vegetable family and have all the amazing fat-burning, cancer-fighting, anti-inflammatory, healthy benefits that broccoli, cauliflower, kale, arugula and cabbage contain. Brussels sprouts' health benefits have been well-studied, and many of the studies have to do with the benefits of this vegetable and its powerful cancer-fighting abilities.

Brussels sprouts provide vital nutrients for the body's detoxification system, its antioxidant system, and inflammatory system, which help prevent chronic diseases and cancer. A healthy diet that includes Brussels sprouts arms your body to effectively fight: bladder cancer, breast cancer, colon cancer, lung cancer, prostate cancer, and ovarian cancer.

Brussels sprouts actually contain omega 3 fatty acids that help fight inflammation as well. About a cup and a half of Brussels sprouts provide about 430 milligrams of plant based omega 3 fatty acid (ALA). And, Brussels sprouts supply antioxidants, including vitamins K, C, E, and A, manganese, quercetin, kaempferol, and more.

The amazing amount of Vitamin K in Brussels sprouts actually fights chronic inflammation. This nutrient helps to regulate our inflammatory response, including chronic inflammation that increases the risk of certain cancers.

Brussels sprouts' anti-inflammatory benefits also help fight obesity, Crohn's disease, inflammatory bowel disease, insulin resistance, irritable bowel syndrome, rheumatoid arthritis, type 2 diabetes, and ulcerative colitis.

Ingredients

- 20-25 small Brussels sprouts
- 4 slices thick-cut (nitrite free) natural bacon, cut into pieces
- 2 tablespoons extra virgin olive oil
- 2 Tbsp butter, melted
- Sea salt and pepper

Directions
Preheat oven to 400 degrees F.
Wash and dry the Brussels sprouts. Trim off the ends of the sprouts, remove the outer leaves, and cut lengthwise in half.

Slice the bacon into small strips and cook until crispy. Remove bacon from the pan. Add extra virgin olive oil, melted butter, Brussels sprouts, bacon, salt, and pepper to bowl and stir to mix well. Spread Brussels sprouts on a large, flat baking sheet or pan. Roast for 20 minutes, or until the sprouts are just fork-tender. Do not overcook! Remove from the oven and serve immediately. Serves 4.

Alternative method: Cook bacon as above. Add halved Brussels sprouts to pan and brown in oven-proof pan for 5-6 minutes. Stir, and add bacon and bake in oven 10-15 minutes till tender.

Open-Face Veggie Sandwich or Wrap

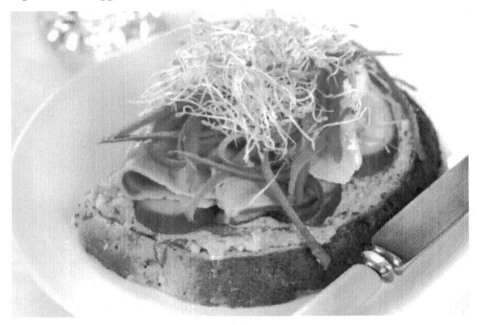

When I am in need of a snack, it seems I always have ingredients for this. There are so many variations on this, you just cannot go wrong! And in the summer when you can get so many of the ingredients fresh and locally grown, life is wonderful!

Ingredients
- 1 slice of whole grain-sprouted Ezekiel bread or whole grain gluten-free bread, toasted gluten-free brown rice tortilla, or for a GRAIN-FREE option, try a sheet of toasted nori
- Avocado
- Tomato
- Red onion sliced thinly
- Sprouts (sunflower sprouts are awesome if you can find them!)
- Lettuce
- Fresh basil leaves
- Other veggies, like zucchini or red pepper
- A slice or two of natural turkey
- Sea salt and pepper if you would like

Directions

Toast bread. Slice up your veggies very thin, except for avocado. When the toast is done, smash and spread half the avocado over the bread. Add a generous amount of sea salt and pepper here, then pile on the meat, onion, tomato, sprouts, etc. Top with a piece of lettuce or sprouts to hold the whole thing together. Serves 1.

(This may be a little messy, so have a plate and a napkin close by!)

Try different variations of veggies and meat on this. The avocado always works well for the base and holds everything together!

Hummus

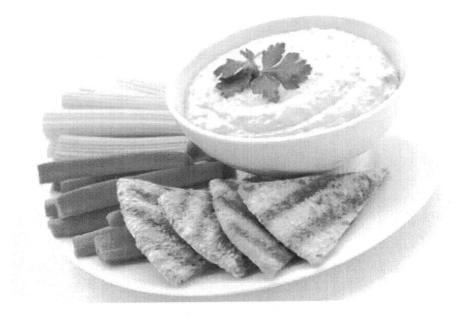

I used to be a vegetarian and ate lots of beans of various types. (I now know this isn't the healthiest diet, so I eat meat now.) Garbanzo beans, or chickpeas, have always been one of my favorites. They are a delicious, filling, healthy super-food.

Hummus is a popular, healthy Middle-Eastern dish made from garbanzos. Garbanzos, or chickpeas, are high in iron, vitamin C, and also have significant amounts of folate (an important B vitamin) and vitamin B6.

The garbanzos make the hummus a good source of protein and fiber, and the tahini, which comes from sesame seeds, is an excellent source of the amino acid methionine, making hummus a complete protein and a perfect snack.

Hummus contains a generous amount of garlic, which has many positive attributes. One of the best health benefits of garlic is its ability to help you lose weight. Garlic is a natural diuretic, and it can help flush out toxins and excess fluid in the body. And, garlic acts as an appetite suppressant—helping you eat less and stimulating your metabolism.

Hummus also contains healthy monounsaturated fats from the extra virgin olive oil. It's important to use a good quality organic extra virgin olive oil, as this makes a huge difference in how the hummus will taste.

The better the quality of extra virgin olive oil, the more antioxidants it contains.

Ingredients
* ¼ cup of sesame tahini (sesame seed paste)
* 1-2 Tbsp of water
* 1 can organic garbanzo beans
* 3 cloves of fresh garlic minced and mashed1 Tbsp extra virgin olive oil
* Juice of 1-2 fresh lemons or limes
* Sprinkle of cayenne pepper or hot pepper flakes
* Handful of fresh parsley

Add-ins: roasted red pepper, sun dried tomatoes, spinach, parsley, cilantro, fresh herbs, or roasted garlic, pitted olives, etc.

Directions
Add the tahini first and slowly add about a tablespoon of water. Blend, then add other ingredients and blend until smooth and creamy. You may need to adjust seasonings after tasting. Hummus should be the consistency of a very thick pudding.

For extra taste and nutrition, try adding roasted red peppers, roasted garlic, ripe olives, hot chili peppers, cilantro, or any of your other favorite fat-burning foods.

Note: Instead of bread or crackers, eat this with sliced organic red, yellow or green bell peppers, cucumbers, tomatoes, and zucchini or other fresh veggies.

Baba Ghanouj

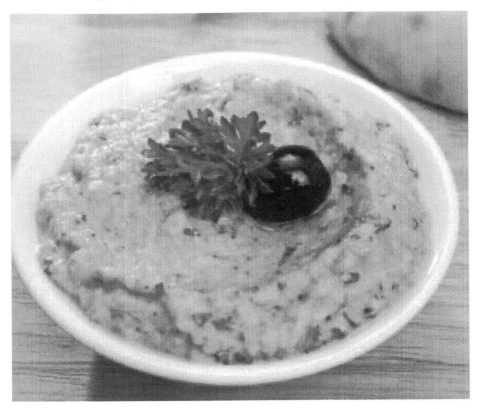

This delicious Middle Eastern dip, similar to hummus, is made from eggplant.

Eggplant not only offers more than its share of vitamins, minerals, and fiber in a low calorie package, but it also has some powerful antioxidants and phyto-nutrients worth mentioning. One of these phytonutrients comes from the dark purple skin, and is called nasunin.

This antioxidant actually protects your cell membranes, especially in the brain, from damage. Cell membranes are made of important fatty acids that protect it from being harmed by invaders like bacteria, viruses and free radicals. Another antioxidant in eggplant, chlorogenic acid, goes to work fighting cancer, bacteria, viruses and fungi, as well as lowering your LDL (bad) cholesterol.

Baba ghanouj, also called baba ghanoush, is a purée of eggplant flavored with tahini (sesame seed paste), lemon juice, garlic and fresh herbs. It is especially tasty with slices of fresh vegetables like cucumbers, carrots, red and green bell peppers and zucchini for dipping.

Ingredients
- 1 large eggplant (about 1 pound), halved lengthwise
- 3 Tbsp sesame tahini
- 1 to 2 cloves garlic, finely chopped
- 2 Tbsp nonfat plain yogurt
- ½ cup parsley leaves, chopped, plus more for garnish
- 1/4 cup lemon juice
- Sea salt to taste
- 1 Tbsp extra virgin olive oil, plus more for garnish

Directions
Preheat oven to 350 degrees F. Place eggplant cut-side down on a foil-lined baking sheet. Prick the skin all over with a fork and bake until soft and collapsed, about 20-30 minutes, depending on its size.

When cool enough to handle, scoop eggplant pulp into a bowl, and discard skin. Add tahini, garlic, yogurt, parsley, lemon juice, salt, and extra virgin olive oil. Mash for a chunky texture, or purée in a food processor, (before adding parsley) for a smooth texture.

Garnish with parsley and drizzle with extra virgin olive oil. Serve with fresh sliced veggies for dipping. Serves 4-6.

Phat Guacamole Deviled Eggs

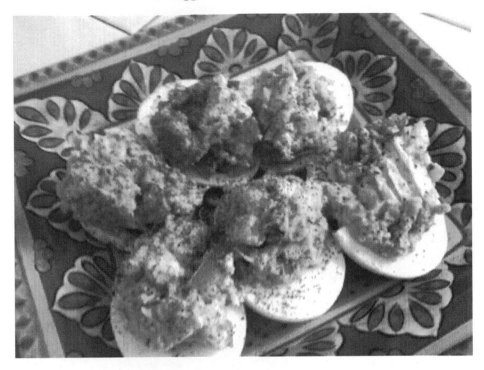

These delicious eggs have guacamole as a healthy addition to the egg yolks. So on top of all the great fat burning benefits you get from eating the eggs and the yolk, you get the healthy fats, vitamins and minerals in the avocado as well.

The healthy fats and other nutrition you get from avocados help your body to maintain proper levels of hormones that help with fat loss and muscle building. The healthy fat in avocados helps control insulin levels and gives your brain a signal that you are satisfied when you eat them, so you eat less.

Avocados contain plenty of oleic acid, a monounsaturated fat that helps lower cholesterol and is helpful in preventing breast cancer and other cancers. One cup of avocado has about a quarter of your required daily amount of folate, or folic acid, a B vitamin that plays an essential role in making new cells by helping to produce DNA and RNA.

This hunger-satisfying low-carb snack will keep your blood sugar stable, replenish and fuel your body with lean, fat-burning nutrition.

Check these out—they are absolutely delicious!

Ingredients
- 4-6 eggs, hard-boiled
- 1 avocado
- 1 clove minced garlic
- ¼ cup finely minced red onion
- 1 small Roma or plum tomato, seeded and finely chopped
- 2-4 Tbsp chopped cilantro
- Frank's Redhot sauce or Tabasco, more or less to taste, depending on its hotness
- 1 tsp lemon or lime juice
- Cilantro, chopped
- Sea salt

Directions
Peel hard-boiled eggs and cut in half length-wise. Gently pop out yolks into a small bowl with avocado, garlic, tomato, onion, hot sauce and lemon juice. Mash yolks and avocado mix together. Season with sea salt, and freshly ground black pepper to taste.

Refill egg whites with the yolk/guacamole mixture, sprinkle with chopped cilantro. Serves 4.

Maximize Your Flat Belly Journey: Get Powerful Fat Loss Secrets From Key Food And Fitness Experts.
http://velocityhousepresents.com/FlatBellyKitchen

Nutty Energy Snack Bombs

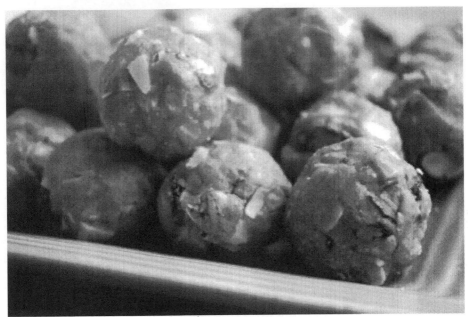

Photo courtesy Isabel ; tisthefood.wordpress.com

These energy snacks are far, far better than most energy bars that you would buy in a store! They not only taste better, but also are WAY healthier for you! And they have only REAL ingredients in them—nothing processed or artificial. And best of all, they contain lots of super fat-burning power!

Several studies have shown that dieters who include reasonable amounts of nuts in their diet actually lose more weight than those who don't eat nuts. Nuts are the perfect fat-burning snack.

Protein and fat in nuts helps you feel full and stops cravings, and won't raise blood sugar, which means they are more likely to be used as energy and will not stimulate your appetite like a starchy or sweet food will.

Nuts help maintain higher levels of fat-burning hormones in your body, as well as helping to control appetite and cravings so that you eat less calories overall, even though you're consuming a high-fat food.

Besides their lean body benefits, nuts are a highly nutritious food to include in your diet.

Most nuts are high in monounsaturated fats, the same type of health-promoting fats as are found in extra virgin olive oil, which have been associated with reduced risk of heart disease and cancer. Nuts also contain polyunsaturated fats, healthy saturated fats, and linoleic acid, another healthy fat that the body utilizes for essential fatty acids.

Nuts contain lots of vitamin E, which works as an antioxidant, and prevents oxidation of LDL cholesterol. Nuts are also chock full of hard-to-get minerals, such as copper, iron, magnesium, manganese, zinc and selenium.

Ingredients
- ½ cup almond butter, peanut butter, or cashew butter
- ½ cup ground flaxseeds
- ½ cup tahini
- ¼ cup pumpkin seeds, walnuts, pecans, almonds, cashews, etc.
- ½ cup grated or shredded unsweetened coconut
- ¼ cup extra virgin coconut oil
- 2 Tbsp cup real maple syrup
- ½ cup dried goji berries, cranberries, cherries, or raisins
- ¼ cup vanilla protein powder (optional)

Combine all ingredients in a medium size bowl, or use a food processor. Roll into balls about the size of a small walnut. These are even better tasting rolled in shredded coconut. Store in refrigerator. Makes about 20 balls.

Experiment with your favorite nuts, dried fruit and nut butters for more varieties of these high-powered snacks.

Berry Delicious

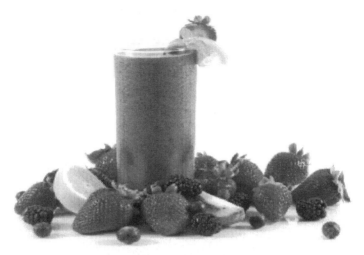

Berries and other fresh or frozen fruits have tremendous antioxidant power, and are high in fiber, and vitamins. The best fruits are organic, and locally grown—if you can find them. Berries are packed with nutrition, and the best ones are goji berries, acai berries, blackberries, and blueberries. If you cannot find fresh fruit, look for organic frozen fruit and berries. Frozen is just as good and will help make your smoothie extra thick and frosty. Avoid commercially grown fruits especially strawberries and peaches, as they are full of pesticides and herbicides and some of the worst things to eat—unless organic.

Ingredients (these are just approximate amounts—no need to measure)
- 1 cup or so of any combination of organic fresh or frozen berries and or cherries
- 1 medium sized banana
- 1-2 Tbsp coconut oil
- 1 Tbsp almond butter, peanut butter or a handful of almonds, walnuts,
- pecans, etc.
- 1 (clean) raw organic egg or protein powder
- 1 cup coconut juice or coconut water
- Sprinkle of cinnamon
- A few ice cubes (optional)

Add all ingredients to blender, and blend until smooth. Enjoy!

Piña Colada Smoothie

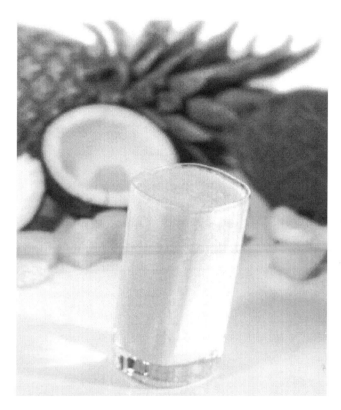

The addition of fresh pineapple lends an anti-inflammatory boost to this smoothie. Pineapple contains bromelain which helps get rid of post-work-out muscle aches and pains, as well as arthritis, and other inflammation.

Ingredients
- 1 medium banana
- 1 cup of fresh pineapple
- 1 cup of coconut milk or 1 cup coconut water
- 1 Tbsp of extra virgin coconut oil
- Protein powder, or 1 raw organic egg (or both)
- Ice cubes (optional)

Add to blender and blend until smooth.

Chocolate Monkey

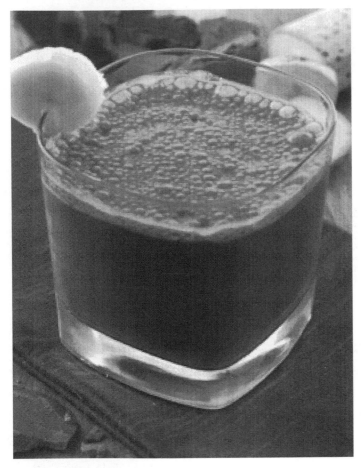

Dark chocolate contains a variety of powerful fat-burning, anti-aging antioxidants, making it excellent for heart and vascular health, and lowering blood pressure as well. Chocolate also helps brain function, and elevates one's mood, raising levels of the feel good hormone, endorphins.

A number of studies show that dark chocolate actually has a very favorable effect on blood sugar levels, as well as diabetes, and decreases inflammation associated with heart disease, dementia, and arthritis.

Dark cocoa appears to contain unique properties that can reduce weight gain, and seems to have appetite suppressing properties. So a nibble of dark chocolate can be a delicious and satisfying sweet treat. When you are choosing chocolate bars, look for the darkest chocolate you can find with the highest percentage of cacao, for maximum health benefits.

Ingredients

- 1 cup of raw organic dairy milk, coconut milk, almond milk or hemp milk
- 2 Tbsp cacao nibs or organic (70% or more) dark chocolate pieces, or organic powdered dark chocolate • 1 banana
- 1 Tbsp of extra virgin coconut oil
- Protein powder (chocolate or vanilla) or 1 raw organic egg or both
- Ice cubes if desired

Blend until smooth.

Pear and Kale Smoothie

The green grapes added to this delightful pear and kale smoothie improve blood circulation and prevent harmful blood clots from forming. And the flavinol, an antioxidant found in the grapes, fights free radicals, repairs tissue in the body and is anti-aging. The oranges provide fresh vitamin C, which helps the body's immune system, protects the blood vessels, and helps prevent wrinkles and keeps the skin looking young.

<u>**Ingredients**</u>
- 1 cup green or red seedless grapes
- 1 large peeled orange
- ½ pear
- 1 large banana
- 1 cup of kale
- ½ cup of water
- Ice cubes

Add all ingredients to blender and blend on high. Add more water if necessary. Makes 2-4 servings. Can be stored in refrigerator or freezer for later use.

Anti-inflammatory Fat-Burning Apple Smoothie

<u>Ingredients</u>
- 8 large kale leaves, stems removed
- 2 small apples
- 2 bananas
- 6 dates
- 1-2 tsp turmeric
- 1 Tbsp (approximately) fresh ginger root, coarsely chopped
- ½ cup water
- Ice cubes if desired

Blend all ingredients on high. Serves 2-4.

Cran-Orange Blast

Cranberries have been used for hundreds of years as a medicine and a poultice for wounds, and we now know that compounds in cranberries have powerful antibiotic effects as well.

While cranberries are best known for helping urinary health, recent studies now suggest that this little red super-berry is beneficial for the gastrointestinal tract, prevents cavities, helps prevent kidney stones and gallstones, aids in recovery from strokes, prevents cancer, lowers LDL (bad) cholesterol, and raises HDL (good) cholesterol. Not bad for one little berry, huh?

These phytochemical powerhouses are packed with five times the antioxidant content of broccoli, and rank higher in antioxidants than most fruits and vegetables!

Several newly discovered compounds in cranberries have also been found to be toxic to cancer cells including lung, cervical, prostate, breast and leukemia cancer cells.

The cranberries in this smoothie are delicious, tart and tangy.

<u>Ingredients</u>
- 1 orange, peeled
- 1 cup of fresh cranberries, or frozen if fresh is not available
- 1 lemon or lime, peeled
- 1 ripe pear
- 2 large collard green leaves or kale, stems removed
- 1 handful organic spinach, large stems removed
- 1 banana
- 1 cup or more of coconut water

Blend all ingredients on high. Serves 2-4.

Mike Geary's Healthy Fat Blend Balsamic Vinaigrette Dressing

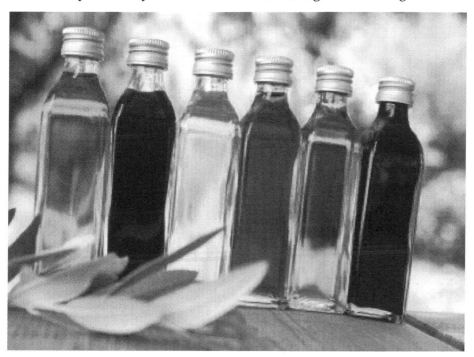

Typical grocery store salad dressings almost always contain refined, processed soybean oil, corn oil and/or canola oil (all VERY unhealthy for you). Many salad dressing try to trick you into believing their products are made with extra virgin olive oil by advertising, "made with extra virgin olive oil" on the front label.

But sad to say, when you actually read the ingredients on the back label, you will find out it contains only a tiny bit of extra virgin olive oil and the rest is usually refined soybean oil, or some other highly processed vegetable oil, which as we know are NOT good for you. On top of that, they may add sugar, corn syrup, corn starch, and chemical preservatives as well.

Don't top your healthy salad with unhealthy junky dressing. Make your own truly healthy salad dressing instead, and you will know exactly what is in it. This great dressing from Mike is as tasty as it is healthy. Pour it on!

Directions

Fill your salad dressing container with these approximate ratios of liquids:

1/3 of salad dressing container filled with balsamic vinegar
1/3 of salad dressing container filled with apple cider vinegar

Fill the remaining 1/3rd of container with equal parts of extra virgin olive oil and "Udo's Choice EFA Oil Blend"

Add just a small touch (approx 1 or 2 teaspoons) of real maple syrup.

Add a little bit of onion powder, garlic powder, and black pepper and then shake the container to mix all ingredients well.

Mike's Note:
The reason I choose to blend the extra virgin olive oil half and half with the Udo's Choice Oil is that they make up for what each lacks. Although extra virgin olive oil is healthy and contains important antioxidants, it is mostly monounsaturated, and is low in the essential fatty acids (EFA's).

The Udo's Choice Oil is higher in unrefined polyunsaturated oils with a good healthy balance of omega 3 to omega 6 fatty acids. There are several variations of the Udo's Choice Oil, and one of them (labeled DHA 3-6-9 Blend) even contains a DHA-rich algae oil blended into the mix along with organic flax oil, coconut oil, evening primrose oil, rice bran oil, oat germ and bran oil, and a few others.

Overall, blending Udo's with extra virgin olive oil makes nearly a perfect oil blend for salad dressings with a great taste and maximum health benefits.

Homemade Ranch Dressing

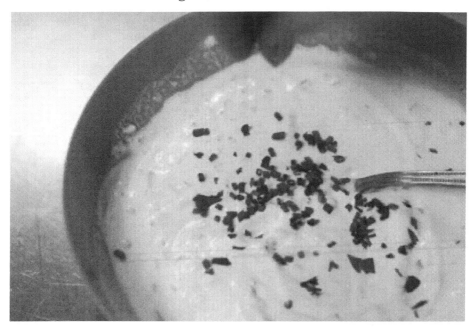

This is a delicious, healthier version of Ranch Dressing with healthy fats and fresh antioxidant charged herbs. This dressing can make a plain green salad exciting, dress up a more elaborate salad, or become a great dip for raw veggies.

Ingredients

- 1/3 cup homemade mayonnaise
- 1/3 cup organic full fat plain or plain Greek yogurt
- 1 1/2 tsp organic apple cider vinegar
- 1/2 tsp honey
- Sea salt and a pinch of cayenne or black pepper to taste
- 1/2 tsp chopped parsley
- 1/4 tsp basil
- 1/8 tsp dill weed
- 3 or 4 spinach leaves
- 2/3 cup extra virgin olive oil, or half and half with Udo's Choice Oil

Directions

Combine all ingredients except oil in blender and puree until smooth. Turn blender on low speed, and while motor is running, carefully pour in oil in a thin stream. When all the oil has been added, turn blender on high and blend a few more seconds to thicken. Store in closed container in refrigerator.

Creamy Avocado Dressing

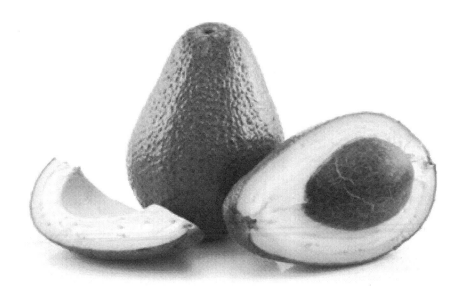

This recipe is easy to make, and you can adjust ingredients to how much you want. Avocados are full of healthy, monounsaturated fats, and bursting with vitamins and phytonutrients.

They add a delicious creamy thickness to dressings—and taste out of this world! Try this on a salad with fresh homegrown tomatoes, or dip cut up veggies into it. I also like it as a sauce over grilled chicken, fish or on a juicy grass-fed burger.

Since avocados tend to turn brown quickly, this dressing generally doesn't keep for more than a day or so, so serve and enjoy immediately.

Ingredients
- • 1 ripe avocado, mashed
- • 1 clove garlic, minced
- • 1⁄4 cup of extra virgin olive oil, or half and half blend of extra virgin olive
- oil and Udo's Choice Oil

- Juice of 1 lemon or lime
- Sea salt and a few sprinkles of red pepper flakes (cayenne) to taste
- Fresh basil, oregano, or thyme, etc., minced finely

Directions
Place all ingredients in a bowl, and mix and mash together thoroughly. Or you can add all to a blender or food processor and mix. Refrigerate in tightly covered container.

Tropical Papaya, Mango and Ginger Salsa (Great on Fish or Chicken!)

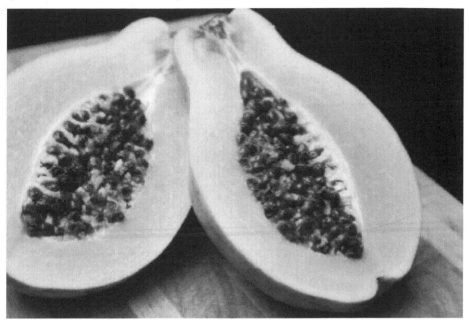

Papayas and mangoes have that luscious, exotic flavor of the tropics, and massive amounts of fat-burning antioxidant nutrients such as carotenes, vitamin C, flavonoids, B vitamins folate and pantothenic acid; potassium, magnesium and fiber.

Papaya also contains the digestive enzyme papain that helps minimize sore muscles and inflammation, arthritis, and allergies. As usual, I like to add a little bit of hot pepper to maximize the fat-burning and metabolism-raising ability. Combined with the cleansing properties of the cilantro, the quercetin in the red onion that helps allergies and inflammation, and the immune enhancing, heart protective benefits of garlic, this is one incredible combination!

A nice variation on this recipe is the addition of fresh pineapple too.

Eat alone and enjoy as a healthy side dish, or serve atop grilled salmon, halibut or chicken.

By Mike Geary, Certified Personal Trainer, Certified Nutrition Specialist
& Catherine Ebeling – RN, BSN

Ingredients

- 1 medium papaya, diced
- 1 mango, diced
- Small bunch of cilantro, minced
- 1 tsp fresh ginger, grated (optional)
- Half of a small red onion, chopped in small pieces
- 1 clove garlic, minced
- Juice of one lime
- Red pepper flakes or half a minced jalapeño or other hot pepper

Directions

Combine all ingredients and enjoy!

Note: When fresh organic peaches are in season, they make a great substitute for mango in this recipe.

Pineapple Salsa

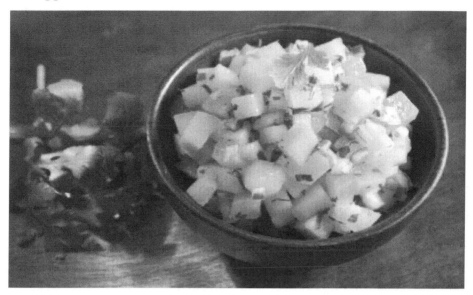

You will love this salsa! It's sweet, hot, tangy, and a perfect addition to grilled salmon, chicken, pork, or just for munching on by itself.

The jalapeños burn fat and increase blood flow, and the cilantro has valuable cleansing properties and can actually help remove toxic metals like mercury from your body.

The pineapple contains a unique ingredient, bromelain. Bromelain is a proteolytic enzyme that helps break down protein, which is why pineapple is known to be a digestive aid. Bromelain is also considered an effective anti-inflammatory, helpful for conditions like arthritis, autoimmune diseases, and sore muscles.

Pineapple is also high in manganese, a mineral that is critical to development of strong bones and connective tissue. A cup of fresh pineapple will give you nearly 75% of the recommended daily amount. It is particularly beneficial to older adults, whose bones tend to become more brittle with age. Fresh pineapple is also high in vitamin C, and because of the bromelain it contains, it has the ability to reduce and break up mucus in the nose and throat. If you have a cold with a cough, add a generous amount of pineapple to your diet.

Maximize Your Flat Belly Journey: Get Powerful Fat Loss Secrets From Key Food And Fitness Experts.
http://velocityhousepresents.com/FlatBellyKitchen

Combined with the anti-inflammatory effects of the onion, the immune enhancing of the garlic and the fat burning of the hot pepper, you can't go wrong with this tasty side dish!

Ingredients
- ½ fresh pineapple, chopped in small pieces
- 1 Roma tomato, chopped
- ½ red onion or several green onions, minced
- 1-2 cloves garlic, minced
- 1 small jalapeño, seeded and ribs removed and minced
- Handful of fresh cilantro, chopped finely
- Juice of one fresh squeezed lime
- Sea salt to taste

Directions
Add all chopped ingredients and stir. Taste for seasoning. Serves 4.

Fresh Tomato Salsa

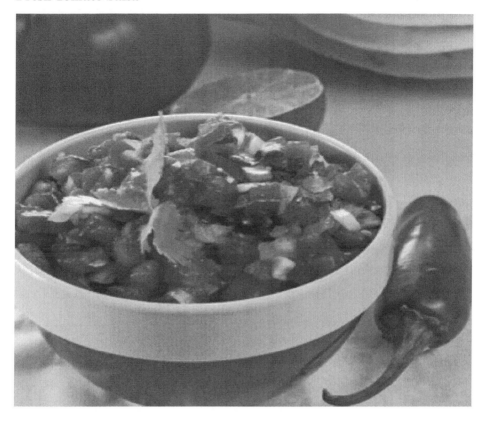

There is nothing better than fresh tomato salsa in the middle of the summer! If you can find the tomatoes at a local farmers' market, at the peak of their ripe- ness and brimming with flavor and fat burning nutrients, this stuff is absolute heaven!

And, the best thing is, you can eat as much as you want of this salsa—there is absolutely nothing in it that will make you fat, and it is loaded with tons of healthy nutrients, like cancer-fighting lycopene, inflammation-busting querce- tin and metabolism-raising capsaicin.

Ingredients are all approximate, and you can adjust according to taste, etc. Good with ANYTHING—on salads, steaks, burgers, grilled chicken or fish, or as an eye-opener with your eggs in the morning—or all by itself with just a fork.

Ingredients
- 4-6 fresh, ripe tomatoes, depending on size, chopped in small pieces
- ½ red onion, minced
- 2 garlic cloves, minced
- 1 jalapeño pepper, ribs and seeds removed, and minced finely
- 1 organic or locally grown green or red bell pepper, chopped in small pieces
- 1 big bunch of cilantro, finely chopped
- Juice of one lemon or lime
- Sea salt

Directions
There are two ways to make this salsa. One method is the chunky version. Just chop all the ingredients and mix together with the lime or lemon juice and sea salt. You can make it extra chunky or use a finer chop.

For a smoother, more pureed version, coarsely chop the veggies and place in a food processor to mix. Process just enough so mixture is smooth, with no large chunks and serve. This will produce a slightly juicier version, so you can drain off some of the excess juice with a colander. Add lemon, lime and salt after draining liquid.

Either way, you will enjoy it immensely! Serves 4 or more.

Basic Soy Teriyaki Marinade

Ingredients
- 1 cup soy sauce
- ½ cup water
- 2 Tbsp of honey or brown sugar
- Juice of one fresh squeezed lemon or lime
- A splash of orange juice (optional)
- 1 Tbsp of fresh grated ginger root
- Fresh ground black pepper or a pinch of cayenne
- 2 garlic cloves
- 2 Tbsp extra virgin olive oil

Balsamic Vinegar Marinade

Ingredients
- ½ cup balsamic vinegar
- ¼ cup extra virgin olive oil or Udo's Choice oil
- 1-2 minced garlic cloves
- ¼ tsp pepper
- Fresh thyme or rosemary, minced

My Favorite Fajita Marinade

While this works great on fajitas, you can use it to marinate beef, chicken or pork anytime for great flavor.

Ingredients
- 1 cup each of gluten-free soy sauce and Worcestershire sauce
- Juice of one lemon or lime
- 1 tsp of cumin powder
- 1 tsp chili powder
- 1-2 garlic cloves, minced
- Generous sprinkle of red pepper flakes

Maximize Your Flat Belly Journey: Get Powerful Fat Loss Secrets From Key Food And Fitness Experts.
http://velocityhousepresents.com/FlatBellyKitchen

Mojo Marinade

This is a power packed, tangy marinade that pairs well with beef, pork, chicken, and fish, but the high acidity makes it easy to over-marinate. I wouldn't marinate for over an hour with this one or meat can become tough.

If you'd like the extra citrus flavor in your meat, add about 5 minutes before done cooking. Just be sure the marinade has thoroughly heated through at medium to high heat to kill any bacteria from the raw meat.

Ingredients:
- Bulb (yes, a whole bulb) of garlic, minced
- 2 tsp salt
- 1 tsp ground black pepper
- 1/2 cup orange juice
- 1/2 cup lime juice
- 1/2 cup lemon juice
- Zest from the citrus
- 2 tsp cumin
- Sprinkle of red pepper flakes

Barbeque Spice Rub

Ingredients
- 3 Tbsp paprika
- 1 Tbsp brown sugar
- 1 Tbsp dried oregano
- 1 Tbsp finely ground coffee
- 1 ½ tsp sea salt
- ½ tsp fresh black pepper

Directions
Coat 2 lbs or so of poultry, meat or seafood with the rub and press gently into the meat to help it stick. (you may want to coat meat with a small amount of extra virgin olive oil first).

Cajun Rub

Ingredients
- 1 Tbsp mustard powder
- 1 Tbsp ground cumin
- 2 tsp celery seeds
- 1 ½ tsp fresh black pepper
- 1 tsp kosher salt
- 1 tsp brown sugar
- 1/8 tsp cayenne pepper

Directions
Coat meat well, cover and store in refrigerator for 2 hours or more.

Spicy Blackened Rub

Ingredients
- ¼ cup paprika
- 3 Tbsp white pepper
- 1 Tbsp cayenne (powdered red pepper)
- 2 Tbsp thyme
- 4 Tbsp garlic powder
- 2-3 Tbsp black pepper
- 1 tsp sea salt

Directions
Rub onto meat and grill or cook over medium-high heat in a cast iron skillet. Spices may be slightly blackened when cooked. You may want to adjust the cayenne pepper and black pepper according to your own tastes. This makes a pretty spicy rub, but remember the hotter the taste the better fat burning properties it has!

Maximize Your Flat Belly Journey: Get Powerful Fat Loss Secrets From Key Food And Fitness Experts.
http://velocityhousepresents.com/FlatBellyKitchen

Jerk Spice Rub

One of my all-time favorites! A delicious sweet and spicy flavor addition. I love this on grilled chicken, along with a pineapple salsa or peanut sauce to go with it. Mmm!!

<u>**Ingredients**</u>
- 1 Tbsp plus 1 tsp dried thyme leaves, crushed
- 1 Tbsp onion powder
- 1 Tbsp turbinado sugar or organic sugar
- 2 tsp rubbed sage
- 2 tsp ground allspice
- 2 tsp black pepper, finely ground
- 1 tsp cayenne pepper
- ½ tsp ground nutmeg
- ½ tsp ground cinnamon

<u>**Directions**</u>
Rub spice mixture on meat and grill or broil.
Note: Cook away from direct heat source, as the slight amount of sugar in this rub tends to burn easily.

Mike Geary's Lean-Body Chocolate Peanut Butter Fudge

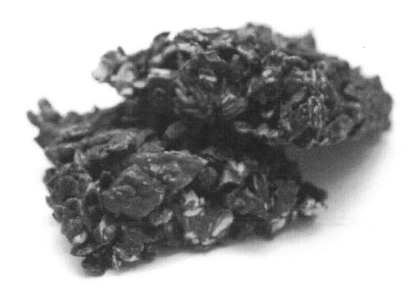

- ¼ cup raw chopped pecans (optional)
- 1 scoop, (about 25 g) protein powder
- 3 Tbsp chia seeds, hemp seeds, and/or flax seeds (optional, but adds crazy amounts of vitamins, minerals, and antioxidants...plus a nutty taste)
- 2 Tbsp rice bran or ground flax seeds (usually only available at health food stores)
- 2 Tbsp whole oats or oat bran
- ½ tsp vanilla extract
- A little natural stevia powder to sweeten (add a small amount to your taste)
- A touch of real maple syrup if you want a more "blended" sweetness flavor

<u>Directions</u>
Start by adding the coconut milk (cans of organic coconut milk are available at most health food stores and possibly even your grocery store) and vanilla extract to a small saucepan on VERY low heat—the lowest heat setting. Break up the extra dark chocolate bar into chunks and add into pot. Add the nut butters and the stevia, and continuously stir until it all melts together into a smooth mixture.

Maximize Your Flat Belly Journey: Get Powerful Fat Loss Secrets From Key Food And Fitness Experts.
http://velocityhousepresents.com/FlatBellyKitchen

Then add the raisins, nuts, seeds, protein powder, oat bran, and rice bran and stir until fully blended. If the mixture becomes too thick or crumbly, just add a small amount more coconut milk. If the mixture seems too wet, keep in mind that it will solidify a good bit once it goes in the fridge.

Spoon/pour the fudge mixture onto some waxed paper in an 8"x 8" baking dish and place in the fridge until it cools and solidifies together (3-4 hours). Cut into squares once firm and place in a closed container or cover with foil in fridge to prevent it from drying out.

Enjoy small squares of this delicious healthy super-food fudge for dessert and for small snacks throughout the day. This is about as good as it gets for a healthy yet delicious treat!

Even though this is a healthier dessert idea that's lower in sugar and higher in nutrition than most sweet treats, keep in mind that it is still calorie dense, so keep your portions reasonable.

Fresh Blackberry or Mixed Berry Tart

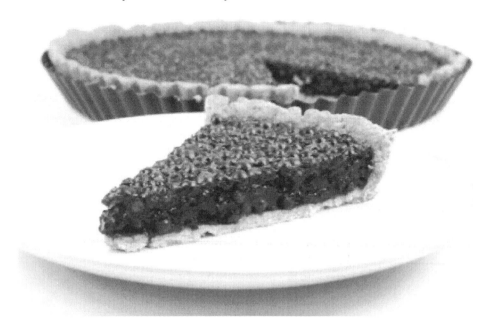

This fabulous fruit tart is bursting with some potent antioxidants, vitamins, minerals and fiber! Eating a variety of fresh berries is one of the best ways to fight aging.

The high-powered antioxidants in the berries protect and smooth your skin and help prevent wrinkles, strengthen your immune system, and fight off cancer and heart disease. Antioxidants also speed up your metabolism, giving you more energy, and helping you burn fat as well!

Berries are a luscious, juicy, sweet treat that fill you up with their healthy fiber and help keep your blood sugar stable as well, meaning you stay in the fat-burning zone.

The crunch, nutty crust is low glycemic and grain free. Nuts are a far better choice than a regular pastry crust of starchy refined flours. And what's more, nuts are full of healthy monounsaturated fats such as *oleic* and *palmitoleic acids*, which help to lower LDL or "bad cholesterol" and increase HDL or "good cholesterol".

Nuts are also a rich source of B vitamins, vitamin E, and minerals including: manganese, potassium, calcium, iron, magnesium, zinc, fluoride and selenium.

Ingredients for Crust
- 1 ¾ cups raw almonds, walnuts or pecans
- 1 Tbsp coconut oil or grass-fed butter
- 5 fresh dates, pitted
- Pinch of nutmeg
- 2 tsp of cinnamon
- Pinch of sea salt
- 1-2 Tbsp raw honey (just enough so that dough will stick together)

Directions for Crust
Finely chop the nuts in a food processor. Add the oil, dates, and spices. Blend together until fine and crumbly. Transfer mixture to a mixing bowl, add honey, and mix to form a dough ball. Add more honey, if needed, so that mixture sticks together.

Grease a 9" pie pan with coconut oil or grass-fed butter, and spread the dough into the bottom of the pan. Bake at 350 degrees F for about 10-12 minutes, until the edges are just beginning to brown.

Ingredients for Filling
- 4-5 cups (around 1 quart) fresh or frozen organic blackberries, cherries, blueberries, strawberries, or raspberries (any combination is great)
- 3 Tbsp raw honey
- 1 ½ Tbsp arrowroot
- 2 Tbsp water, or juice if using frozen berries

Directions for Filling
If you are using frozen berries make sure they are completely thawed, so they do not get too juicy and dilute the filling.

Add 2 cups of the berries along with the arrowroot in a blender. Add 2 Tbsp water or berry juice. Blend into a puree. Cook puree in small saucepan with honey over medium heat, stirring constantly for about 3-4 minutes. It will become clear as it thickens.

Remove from heat and cool slightly. Add remainder of berries and fill shell. Refrigerate, covered at least 3 hours. Make sure it is covered so it doesn't pick up moisture from the refrigerator.

For an extra special treat, top with REAL whipped cream.

REAL Whipped Cream Topping
Whip a half pint of organic heavy cream with an electric mixer in a metal bowl until soft peaks form. Add a touch of stevia and a splash of vanilla and mix. Keep chilled until ready to use.

Raw Apple Pie

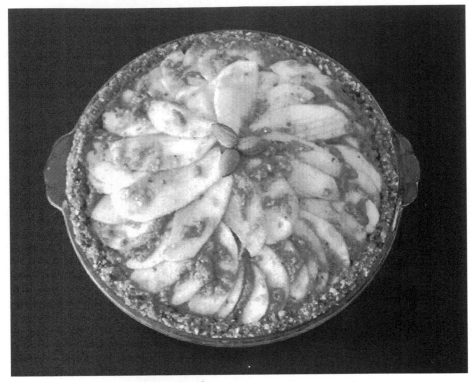

Photo courtesy of www.vegansweettooth.com

We have all heard the saying, "An apple a day, keeps the doctor away." Do you know why? Apples may not be as glamorous and trendy as some of the latest superfoods, but they contain some pretty mighty ingredients that safeguard your health.

Apples contain phloridzin and boron to strengthen bones. The quercetin in apples helps allergy and asthma symptoms, protects against Alzheimer's disease, liver and lung cancer; and the pectin and fiber in the skin help to maintain a healthy digestive tract, lower the risk of colon cancer, keep blood sugar stable, and aids in weight loss.

Conventional apples are loaded with pesticides, so be sure to choose organic apples. But do eat the skin of organic apples whenever you can. The skin contains many of the most powerful antioxidants in apples—as well as the fiber—

and eating it raw is the best way to preserve and protect the antioxidants and the active enzymes as well.

This crust is made of a rich, crunchy blend of pecans and walnuts which is not only high in healthy fats, vitamins and minerals, but also delightfully delicious as well!

Crust Ingredients
- ¼ cup pecans
- ¼ cup walnuts
- 5 or 6 medjool dates-pitted
- 1 Tbsp coconut oil
- Pinch of sea salt

Directions
Pulse the nuts in a food processor until they form a coarse meal. Spread crust mixture thinly in a 9" pie pan and press down with fingers. For a thicker crust, double the crust ingredients. Store crust in refrigerator until ready to fill with apples.

Filling Ingredients
- 1 orange, peeled and seeded
- 1 apple, peeled and cored
- 1 cup pitted dates
- 2 tsp cinnamon
- ¼ tsp nutmeg
- 4-5 apples, peeled, cored, and sliced thinly

Directions
Process the orange and one of the apples in the food processor until pureed. Add dates, cinnamon and nutmeg, and process again until smooth.

Place the sliced apples into a large bowl, pour the fruit and spice mixture over it, and carefully toss until apple slices are all thoroughly coated. Layer the apple slices into the prepared crust. Serve immediately or refrigerate for later! Serves 6-8.

Maximize Your Flat Belly Journey: Get Powerful Fat Loss Secrets From Key Food And Fitness Experts.
http://velocityhousepresents.com/FlatBellyKitchen

Dairy-Free Pralines 'N Cream Ice Cream

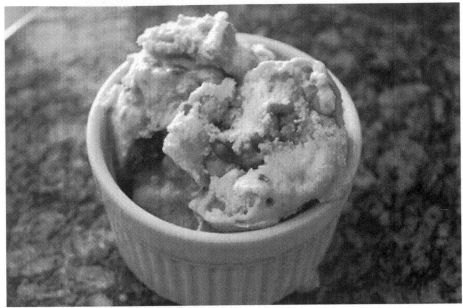

Photo courtesy of http://www.bakedbyjen.com

This recipe contains rich and creamy coconut milk instead of cream from a cow. Coconut milk contains a good-for-you type of saturated fat made up of *medium chain triglycerides*. This fat is immediately utilized as an energy source, for long term energy, helping you burn fat in the process.

Coconut milk also contains an ingredient called lauric acid, which strengthens your immune system, and fights off pathogens like bacteria, viruses and fungi. And the fats in coconut milk help make your skin soft and smooth, and your hair shiny as well. Considering all the healthy benefits of the fat in coconut milk, always get the 'full fat' type of coconut milk, not the low fat kind.

Pecans add a delicious nutty crunch, but you can always try other nuts as well like cashews, almonds, or mixed raw nuts.

This recipe is courtesy my friend Kieba in Hawaii, where she conducts a body, mind, and spirit fitness boot camp. She is an expert chef and creates all sorts of delicious dishes for her boot campers, using raw, whole ingredients.

266

Praline Ingredients

- 1 cup chopped pecans
- 5 Tbsp maple syrup or raw honey
- Dash nutmeg
- Dash sea salt
- 1 tsp of cinnamon

Directions

Mix all ingredients and spread in a thin layer on a baking sheet and bake at 300 degrees F or about 20 minutes or until crispy.

Vanilla Ice Cream Ingredients

- 1 cup coconut milk (full-fat)
- 1 cup raw dairy milk or almond milk
- ½ to ¾ cup young coconut meat (optional)
- 1 Tbsp coconut oil
- ¼ cup raw honey or maple syrup
- ½ tsp pure vanilla extract

Directions

Puree ice cream ingredients in a blender or food processor until smooth and freeze 4 hours or more. Remove from freezer and puree again and fold in praline pieces. You can also use a regular ice-cream maker to freeze and thicken this dessert. Fold in pralines just before serving. Enjoy!

Maximize Your Flat Belly Journey: Get Powerful Fat Loss Secrets From Key Food And Fitness Experts.
http://velocityhousepresents.com/FlatBellyKitchen

Dairy-Free Coconut Cream Ice Cream

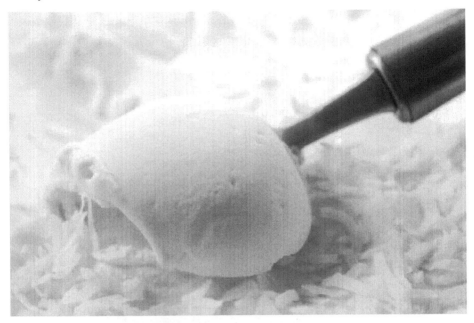

While too much of anything can be bad, this ice cream is made with ultra healthy, creamy (full fat) coconut milk. Coconut milk is a far better choice than conventional milk from cows, and although it is slightly higher in calories, it is a better fat-burning food. The medium chain triglycerides in the fat not only raise metabolism, but are converted immediately to energy, instead of being stored as body fat.

The fat in coconut milk also contains lauric acid, a saturated fat that is good for cholesterol levels because it increases the amount of HDL (good) cholesterol. Lauric acid is also anti-cancer, anti-viral, kills germs, and is good for the brain as well.

Coconut milk is also full of other nutrients, including protein, B and C vitamins, and manganese which helps maintain stable blood sugar levels. It contains copper and iron to help skin and blood vessels stay smooth and flexible, calcium and phosphorus to strengthen bones, magnesium to help muscles and nerves stay relaxed, selenium, a powerful antioxidant, potassium, which helps to balance out the body's electrolytes, as well as zinc for wound healing, muscle growth, and testosterone production.

Enjoy this healthy dessert that is good for your body!

Ingredients

- ½ cup or more of unsweetened coconut cream/milk (the full fat kind)
- 1 tsp pure vanilla extract
- 2 tsp cinnamon
- Tiny pinch of sea salt
- Small amount of Stevia for sweetness, or raw honey or maple syrup, if you prefer

Directions

Mix ingredients in food processor or blender and pour into ice cream maker and freeze, according to directions. If you do not have an ice cream maker, pour into ice cube trays and freeze 4 or more hours. Remove from freezer about 15 minutes before serving and puree again in food processor or blender, and serve.

This is extra good sprinkled with chopped nuts or toasted, unsweetened shredded coconut.

Fresh Strawberry Pie

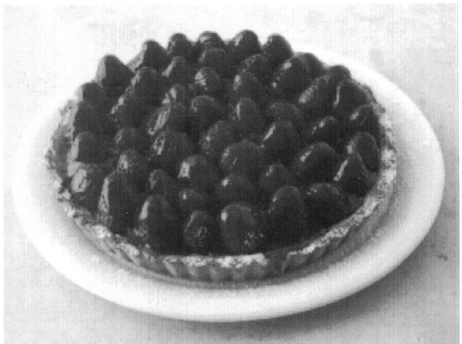

The best tasting pie is made from locally grown strawberries at the height of the strawberry season, which for many of us, is in late spring or early summer. Of course you can always find strawberries in the grocery store pretty much year 'round, but for berries bursting with sweet and juicy flavor, look for locally grown strawberries.

Always buy organic strawberries whenever possible. Conventionally raised strawberries from those huge commercial farms contain loads of pesticides and toxic chemicals that you can't wash off. Conventional strawberries are at the top of the most highly sprayed produce.

Strawberries, like other berries, are a great source of a type of antioxidants, called 'phenols'. One of the phenols in strawberries is what gives them their deep red color. This phenol protects your cells, and prevents free radical damage in the body's organ systems. These unique antioxidants make them heart healthy, cancer preventative, and anti-inflammatory, all in one sweet little juicy package.

Ingredients for Crust
- 1 ½ cup finely crushed* organic almonds or almond meal
- 3 Tbsp melted virgin coconut oil, or grass-fed butter
- 2 Tbsp pure maple syrup
- Pinch of sea salt

Preheat oven to 350 degrees F. Melt coconut oil on stove if it's not already liquid (usually liquid at room temperature). Add maple syrup and crushed almonds into the melted coconut oil and mix well. Then simply use fingertips or another pie pan to press the crust mixture evenly into shape in pan. Bake crust 8 to 10 minutes. Remove the crust from the oven and set aside in the refrigerator.

*Almonds can be crushed in food processor or in plastic bag with a rolling pin

Ingredients for Filling
- 2 pints of organic strawberries, sliced in half
- 1 ½ Tbsp coconut oil
- ½ cup shredded unsweetened coconut (optional)
- 2-4 Tbsp of (full-fat) coconut milk
- 1 tsp pure vanilla extract
- Stevia or raw honey to taste

Directions for Filling
Mix ingredients together and pour into crust. Chill in refrigerator 1-2 hours, and serve topped with fresh berries. Serves 4-8.

*Note: If you would like to indulge in a little whipped cream, make the REAL stuff by purchasing a half pint of organic heavy cream. Whip with an electric mixer in a metal bowl until soft peaks form. Add a touch of Stevia, and a splash of vanilla and mix. Keep chilled until ready to use.

Maximize Your Flat Belly Journey: Get Powerful Fat Loss Secrets From Key Food And Fitness Experts.
http://velocityhousepresents.com/FlatBellyKitchen

Coconut Milk Flan

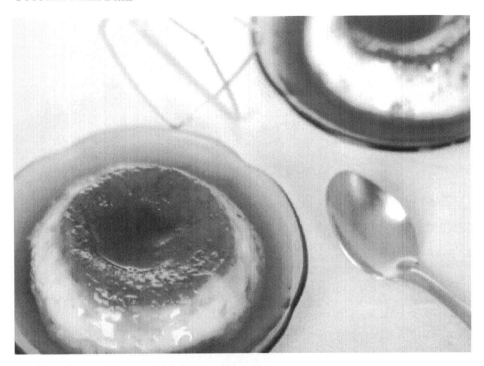

Sweet treats tend to be not only full of calories, but have the unfortunate downside of providing mostly empty calories. But you can have sweet treats that have lots of health benefits too. You will love this one!

The fat in the coconut milk is the single best source of medium chain triglycerides. Why does that matter? This type of healthy fat gets burned immediately for energy. It also boosts your metabolism and helps your body burn fat more easily for energy.

Besides its fat-burning and energy-promoting abilities, coconut oil possesses other great health benefits for your body as well. Coconut oil is also rich in lauric acid, which boosts immunity and destroys harmful bacteria and viruses in the body.

The saturated fat in coconuts is great for your heart, your skin, your hair and your brain as well. Enjoy this dessert and know you are doing good things for your body and health!

Ingredients

- 3 Tbsp raw sugar
- 1 15 oz. can of full-fat, organic coconut milk
- 5 organic, free-range eggs
- 2-3 Tbsp of pure maple syrup
- 1 tsp of real vanilla extract
- 3 ounces of unsweetened shredded coconut for topping (optional)

Directions

Pre-heat the oven to 325 degrees F. Fill a teapot with 2-3 cups water and heat to a simmer.

In saucepan, heat the sugar until it melts and is a golden brown liquid. Pour sugar mixture into a 9" glass pie plate.

Combine all the rest of the ingredients in a large bowl and mix with mixer. Pour into pie plate, and place inside a larger baking dish that is at least 2 inches deep. Then pour the hot water in the space surrounding the pie pan—allowing the liquid to reach about halfway up the sides. Bake about 40 to 45 minutes, or until the flan is set (when a knife comes out clean from the center).

For the topping—line a baking sheet with parchment paper and bake raw, shredded coconut in the same 325 degrees F oven for about 5 to 7 minutes. Remove the toasted coconut once it's lightly browned, and sprinkle on top of flan. Serves 4-5.

Mike 's Lean-Body Recipe: Pumped-Up Pumpkin Mix

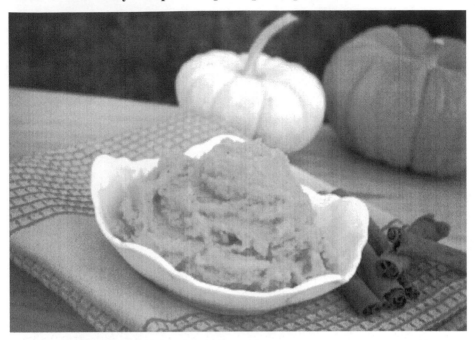

If you like pumpkin pie, you'll love this nutrient-dense, antioxidant-rich, protein-packed treat!

Pumpkins are a rich source of beta carotene and vitamin A, vitamin C, magnesium, potassium, zinc, and fiber which benefit your eyes, skin, immune system, bones, digestion, and heart health. It is also rich in anti-inflammatory compounds, and contains l-trytophan, which helps you sleep and feel calmer. The fiber in pumpkin fills you up without adding tons of calories (unless you're eating pumpkin pie!).

It's funny, but whenever someone sees this little concoction, they say it tastes way better than it looks! I know it's a little "out there", but give it a shot...it tastes like pumpkin pie filling, but tastier, and better for you!

This recipe makes 5-6 servings (I like to split into 5-6 containers to have a quick healthy mid-meal each day).

Ingredients

- Two 15 oz cans of pure 100% organic pumpkin
- One 15 oz container of ricotta cheese (grass-fed if you can find it)
- One 32 oz container of vanilla yogurt
- One scoop (about 25 grams) of vanilla (grass-fed, cold processed, stevia-sweetened) protein powder.
- 3/4 cup raisins or currants
- 3/4 cup chopped walnuts or pecans
- ¼ cup chia seeds and/or hemp seeds
- ¼ cup rice bran
- Cinnamon to season to taste (1/2 to 1 tsp works well)
- A little stevia (natural non-caloric sweetener)—only if it needs a little more sweetness for your taste.

Directions

Mix everything together in a huge bowl and split into 5-6 containers (approx 16 oz containers work well), and you've got a quick healthy snack, or dessert for each weekday. Adjust the quantities of the ingredients if you want fewer calories or more calories per meal.

This would be a big serving for smaller females, so adjust the quantities a little bit lower. For bigger guys, this meal size should be fairly satisfying.

If you like these unique healthy meal ideas, there are 84 other Lean-Body meal ideas included in the Truth about Six Pack Abs program.

Resource Links

U.S. Wellness Meats: http://www.grasslandbeef.com

Steviva: http://www.steviva.com

The Nutrition Investigator, Mike Geary, Discusses Real Nutrition for a Healthy Lean Body: http://www.truthaboutabs.blogspot.com

TruthAboutAbs.com: http://www.truthaboutabs.com

Prograde, krill oil and fish oil supplements: http://www.natural.getprograde.com

BioTRUST: http://www.natural.biotrust.com

Dale's Raw Foods: http://www.dalesrawfoods.com

A Campaign for Real Milk: http://www.realmilk.com

VitalChoice: http://www.vitalchoice.com

Cat's Kitchen Recipes: http://simplesmartnutrition.com

Simple Smart Nutrition: http://www.simplesmartnutrition.com

Avalanche Ski Training: http://www.avalancheskitraining.com

BusyManFitness.com: http://www.busymanfitness.com

About the Authors

Catherine Ebeling RN BSN

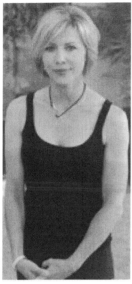

Catherine (Cat) Ebeling is an RN with a Bachelor of Science in Nursing, with a background in physical therapy and over twelve years in the fitness business.

After learning that she had several food allergies at the age of 20, as well as celiac disease–a serious autoimmune disease of the GI tract in which the body attacks the digestive system, she set out to look for solutions. Undiagnosed celiac disease can lead to severe malnutrition, osteoporosis, anemia and many other serious diseases, including cancer.

Not willing to sit around waiting for her health to deteriorate, she studied every nutrition and diet book available in search of the answers to her health problems.

Cat has had more than thirty years of intense study in diet, nutrition, disease and natural alternatives to drugs. As a part of the medical community, it was clear that there was a lot of ignorance among doctors and her peers regarding nutrition and health, so she often became a resource for both doctors, other nurses, and patients for their dietary concerns.

Through the study of diet and health, as well as her work as a fitness professional, she has learned tried and true ways to lose weight, look great, feel young and have tons of energy.

This "simple, smart, nutritional" approach has created real results for many people.

In addition, she has helped many people overcome their health issues and avoid harmful medications and the resulting negative side effects.

Catherine graduated Magna Cum Laude with a BS in Nursing ('05) from St. Louis University, a prestigious medical and scientific university. She also has a Bachelor's Degree in Marketing from Ball State University in Indiana. She is certified as a Personal Trainer by the American Council on Exercise.

As a mother of 20, 19 and 17 year old children, she had to fight to lose weight after having children, and now is back to the size she was in high school and every bit as fit. Cat has been an athlete since she was a child, participating in track as a sprinter and hurdler, and also gymnastics and cheerleading. Throughout her active adulthood, she has pursued many activities including running, weight lifting, aerobics, water skiing, and snow skiing. She now races mountain, cyclocross and road bikes against women half her age, and often wins.

Cat attributes her success in athletics as well as her youthful, healthy outlook on life to a healthy diet and exercise. For more great tips on diet, health and delicious fat burning recipes, see her website http://www.simplesmartnutrition.com/ and subscribe to "Cat's Kitchen", the online e-newsletter and get the inside scoop on what's really in the food you eat, plus get more great healthy, no-grain recipes everyone will love.

Cat teaches healthy cooking seminars, and is a health and wellness consultant for many companies. Cat offers corporate wellness solutions to many of the most troubling (and expensive) health conditions including diabetes, weight loss, heart disease and cancer. In addition she is a health and wellness coach for individuals, and helps them achieve success in their health and weight loss goals. For more information, email Cat at caebeling@gmail.com.

Mike Geary

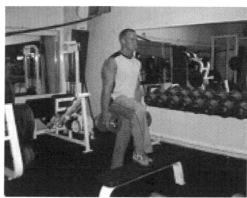

Mike has been a Certified Nutrition Specialist and Certified Personal Trainer for almost 10 years now. Mike has been studying nutrition and exercise for almost 20 years, ever since he was a young teenager. Mike is currently 36 and moved from New Jersey (growing up in the Philadelphia area) to the beautiful mountains of the Colora- do Rockies 5 years ago.

Mike now enjoys skiing almost every day during the winter in Colorado and Utah, and spends a lot of time mountain biking, hiking, golfing, and enjoying other outdoor activities and sports.

Mike is an avid adventurist and in the last several years, has done:

- 3 skydiving jumps (2 of them from 17,000 feet in Colorado)

- 4 whitewater rafting trips including some of the most extreme Class 5 rapids in North America in the well-known Gore Canyon

- Piloting an Italian fighter plane over the desert of Nevada (wow, what a blast!)

- Taking part in a "Zero-Gravity Flight" where you actually experience weightlessness and float around the airplane cabin (the same training given to astronauts)

- Heli-skiing in Chile

- Scuba diving the Silfra Ravine in Iceland in 34-degree F water and 300-feet visibility underwater.

- Snowmobiling and hiking on a glacier that overlies a volcano in Iceland

- Riding Porsche powered dune buggies through the entire length of the

Baja Peninsula of Mexico with 25 high level business owners and CEOs, including Jesse James of West Coast Choppers fame

- Ziplining over canyons and forests in the Rocky Mountains, Costa Rica, and Mexico

- Cruising the entire Caribbean

- Traveling through Nicaragua, Spain, Belize, Costa Rica, Mexico, Iceland, Chile, the Bahamas, Jamaica, Cayman Islands, Turks & Caicos, Trinidad & Tobago, and all over the US/Canada.

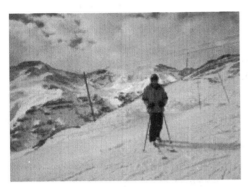

In the last 5 years, Mike has become the best-selling author of the famous *Truth about Six Pack Abs* program with over 439,000 readers currently in 163 countries, and a subscriber base of over 655,000 subscribers worldwide to Mike's Lean-Body Secrets online e-newsletter.

If you don't already receive Mike's weekly Lean-Body Secrets e-newsletter, make sure to sign up here for FREE so you don't miss out on all of Mike's unique fat-burning recipes, crazy workout combinations, and tons more tips to help you live lean and healthy for life!

Mike's *Truth About Six Pack Abs* program has also been translated currently into Spanish, German, and French:
German version: http://www.flacherbauch.com/
Spanish version: http://www.PierdaGrasaAbdominal.com
French version: http://www.toutsurlesabdos.com/

BIBLIOGRAPHY

Bell Muzaurieta, Annie. "Farmed Fish Might Be Unhealthy: New Research Shows Popular Farmed Fish Might Adversely Affect Your Heart Health." *The Daily Green*. May 2008. Hearst Communcations. 07/15/09. http://www.thedailygreen.com/healthy-eating/eat-safe/farmed-tilapia-health-effects-44071408#ixzz0LMdStrCV&C

Dolson, Laura. "Green Leafy Vegetables—Nutritional Powerhouses,." *About.com*. June 2008 About.com, 06/15/09.http://lowcarbdiets.about.com/od/lowcarbsuperfoods/a/greensnutrition.htm

Dolson, Laura. "Eat Your Greens! How to Cook Greens, Types of Greens, Recipes, Cooking Tips,." *About.com*. August 2008. About.com. 06/15/09 http://lowcarbdiets.about.com/od/cooking/a/greensrecipes.htm

Ellison, M.Sc., Shane. "Fat for Energy and Raw Athletic Power."*U.S. Wellness Meats Newsletter*, September 15, 2007.U.S. Wellness Meats, 2007.05/13/09 http://www.uswellnessmeats.com/newsletter_archive/newsletter/2007/September_16_2007_Newsletter.html

Ellison, M.Sc., Shane. "Artificial Sweetner Explodes Internally." *The People's Chemist*.2008. The People's Chemist.com 03/07/09 http://www.thepeopleschemist.com/view_learning.php?learning_id=14

Ephraim, RD, CCN, Rebecca. "Aspartame: Diet-astrous Results." *Wise Traditions in Food, Farming and the Healing Arts*. 06 2000. Weston A. Price Foundation. 06/06/09. http://www.trit.us/modernfood/aspartame.html

"Food Democracy, Fish: Fresh vs. farmed, what you need to know." *Food Democracy*. May 2008.http://fooddemocracy.wordpress.com/2008/05/20/fish-fresh-vs-farmed-what-you-need-to-know/

Gates, Donna. "The 20 health benefits of real butter."*Body Ecology Diet*. 2009. Bodyecology.com. 02/06/09. http://www.bodyecology.com/07/07/05/benefits_of_real_butter.php

"Health Benefits of Nuts, the Snack that Benefits Your Health."*The Healthier Life*. August 2003. Agora Lifestyles. 05/05/09 http://www.thehealthierlife.co.uk/natural-health-articles/nutrition/health-benefits-of-nuts-00841.html

Jonsson, Randolph. Raw-milk-facts.com. 2004. White Tiger construction. 06 07 2009 http://www.raw-milk-facts.com/

Lipinski, Lori. "Milk: It Does a Body Good? It all depends on where it comes from, doesn't it?." *Wise Traditions in Food, Farming and the Healing Arts, the quarterly magazine of the Weston A. Price Foundation*. April 2003. Weston A. Price Foundation.05 07 2009.http://www.westonaprice.org/transition/dairy.html

Masterjohn, Chris. "On the trail of the elusive X-factor." *Weston A. Price Foundation Wise*

By Mike Geary, Certified Personal Trainer, Certified Nutrition Specialist
& Catherine Ebeling – RN, BSN

Traditions in Food, Farming and the Healing Arts. Spring, 2007. Weston A. Price Foundation.06/10/ 09 http://www.westonaprice.org/basicnutrition/vitamin-k2.html

Mercola, Joseph. "Corn Caused Widespread Disease Among Some Native Americans." *Mercola.com.* March 06, 2000. Accessed 06/10/09.http://articles.mercola.com/sites/articles/archive/2000/06/03/corn-part-one.aspx

Starr Hull, Dr. Janet. *Aspartame Dangers Revealed.* 2006. Dr. Janet Starr Hull. 10 June 2009 http://www.sweetpoison.com/

Stier , Ken. "Fish Farming's Growing Dangers." *Time Magazine.*19 09 2007. Time Magazine. May 15, 2009. http://www.time.com/time/health/article/0,8599,1663604,00.html

Thomas Cohen , Sally Fallon. "Fight the Pasteurization Myth." *Weston A. Price Foundation Wise Traditions.*1999. Weston A. Price Foundation. 10 June 2009 http://www.westonaprice.org/basicnutrition/vitamin-k2.html

"The Welfare of Cattle in Beef Production; A Summary of the Scientific Evidence A Farm Sanctuary Report." *Farm Santuary.* 2009. 01 07 2009. http://www.farmsanctuary.org/mediacenter/beef_report.html

Winston Craig, MPH, PhD, RD. "Health Benefits of Green Leafy Vegetables Greens—A Neglected Gold Mine." *Vegetarianism and vegetarian nutrition.* June 23 2009 http://citationmachine.net/index2.php?reqstyleid=1&reqsrcid=14&mode=form&more=&source_title=Web%20Document&source_mod=&stylename=MLA